# HEALTH

## Overcoming Fatigue & Chronic Illness

### By

### Jonathan Troy Hull

www.OvercomeIllness.net

www.facebook.com/overcomeillness

# HEALTH

## Overcoming Fatigue & Chronic Illness

### Jonathan Troy Hull

Copyright © March, 2011 Jonathan T. Hull. No part of this book may be reproduced or transmitted without written permission of the author.

This book is intended solely for educational and informational purposes and not as personal medical advice. Please consult a health care professional if you have any questions about your health.

Cover (front): By author. Depiction of cave art, Algeria, 3,000 BC
(back): Photo by Jon A. Hull, Kenya, 1979

For information about special discounts for bulk purchases, please visit online:
www.OvercomeIllness.net

ISBN 978-0-615-46170-0

For those who struggle with chronic illness

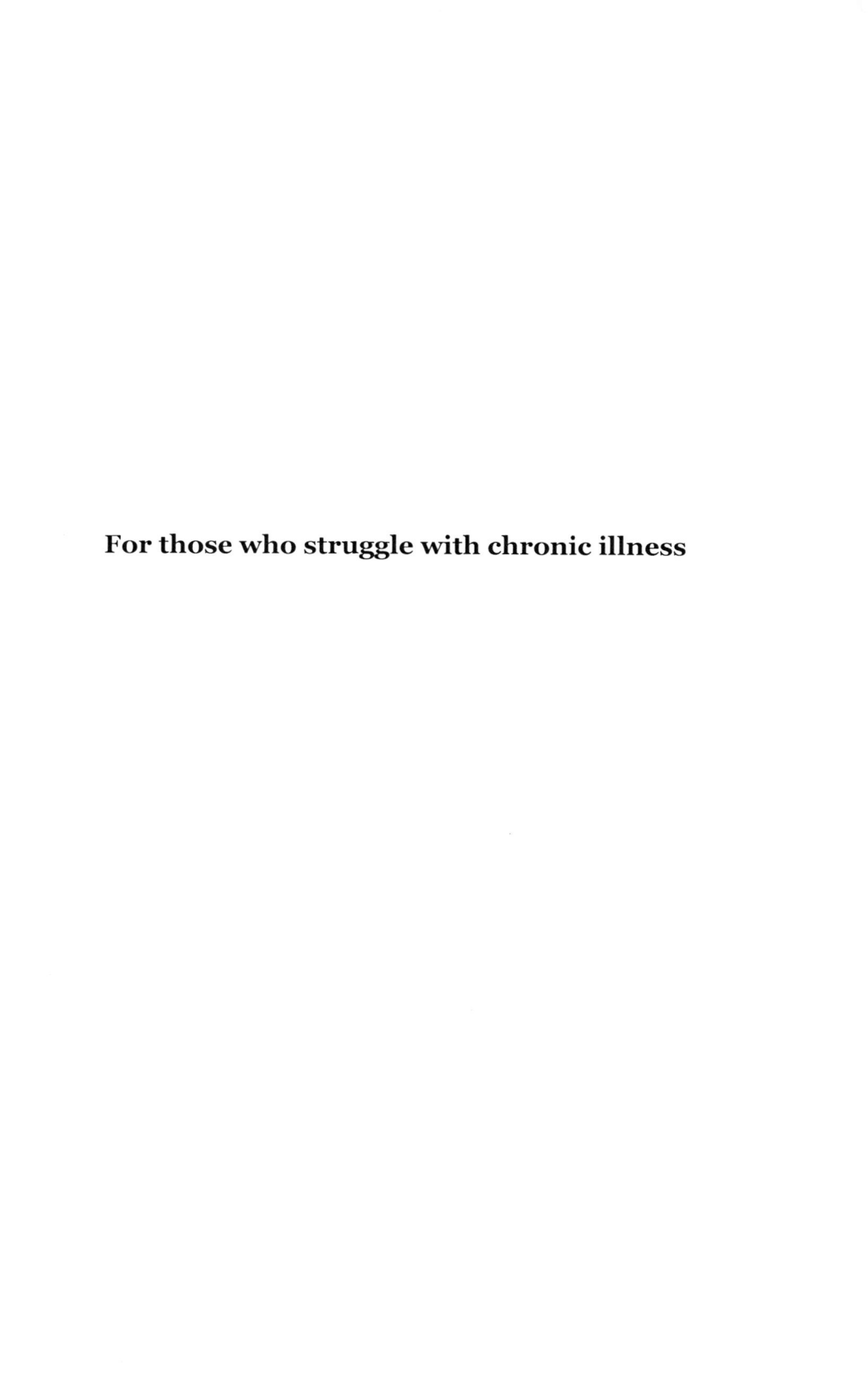

*"Fall down seven times, stand up eight"*

*- Japanese proverb*

## *Acknowledgements*

Special thanks to Nancy Evans for donating her time and skills as a writer and professional editor on the subject of health. This book would not be what it is without her helpful suggestions and keen insight.

Thanks to my family and friends for supporting me in this endeavor and to my son, Jonah, for brightening my life.

# Contents

| | |
|---|---|
| Why read this book?....................................................... | i |
| How this Guide is Organized......................................... | iii |
| Introduction and Disclaimer........................................... | 1 |
| 1. Dreams Deferred....................................................... | 5 |
| 2. Answers..................................................................... | 18 |
| 3. A Crash Course in Nutrition..................................... | 42 |
| 4. Active Digestion (AD) and Passive Digestion (PD)... | 48 |
| 5. A Five-Part Approach to Recovering from CFS and Chronic Illness ............................................................. | 66 |
| 6. The Natural Diet ...................................................... | 78 |
| 7. Meal Ideas to get Started ......................................... | 88 |
| 8. Healing on Restricted Diets ..................................... | 97 |
| 9. The End Game ......................................................... | 100 |
| 10. Health Misunderstandings and Myths .................. | 102 |
| 11. Recovering from other Chronic Illnesses through the Natural Diet and Lifestyle ................................. | 112 |
| About the Author............................................................ | 142 |

## *Why Read this Book?*

There are many books and ideas out there on health and chronic illness. Having spent a number of years scouring bookstores and the internet as well as talking to healthcare professionals of all kinds, I eventually realized that no one else had the answer to what was causing my own fatigue issues. With no other choice, I decided to figure it out on my own and the results of that search are encapsulated in this guide.

In short, I've written this book to help empower people to take control of their own health, and thereby save time and money on unnecessary doctor visits, expensive and ineffective supplements, and potentially harmful medications or surgical procedures.

Some of the things you will find here include:

- A new explanation for Chronic Fatigue Syndrome (CFS) that I have not come across anywhere else to date.

- New ways of understanding digestion that can empower those with digestive problems.

- Detailed descriptions of how to prepare foods and drinks and how to act on your hunger signals in order to manage and overcome chronic fatigue and rebuild your overall health.

- A theory for how most chronic diseases stem from the same cause, and how to overcome them.

I've done my best to not burden the reader with excessive information. My goal in writing this book is simply to share what I've learned and the models I've come up with, and to empower as broad an audience as possible with information and insight that might help improve one's quality of life.

## *How this Guide is Organized*

The first four chapters provide a background to the philosophy and science of what I believe to be the path back to health from a state of compromised digestion-induced illness and chronic fatigue. In chapter one, I describe how my own mysterious symptoms of fatigue came about, marking the beginning of my journey back to good health.

Chapter two introduces the details of my theory for one possible cause of chronic fatigue and how it ties into a broader picture of health in general. While it may not be the only answer, it's the only one I've been able to come up with that seems to make sense in both theory and practice. Chapter two ties in with chapters three and four before the explanation comes full circle. If these chapters seem a little heavy or complicated, just know that things will start coming together in relation to chronic illness in general in chapter five. I realize there are a lot of concepts which may seem complicated for those without a strong science background, so I encourage you to read it at a comfortable pace in order to fully "digest" the information.

I would classify chapter five as the "meat" of this guide. It pulls together five major concepts under a single umbrella, including the "answer" to fatigue that I explain in the first four chapters. I refer to this umbrella concept as the "Natural Diet and Lifestyle," which I believe can mitigate and reverse chronic diseases of all kinds.

Towards the end of the guide I talk about "health myths," of which there are really too many to count. From various cure-all supplements to strange diets that tout the incredible curing potential of only one or two ingredients...the number of advertised ways of recovering from illness are as widespread as the number of quacks looking to make a few dollars.

I end the book with specific examples of how I believe all chronic illnesses are linked and how the cure to these illnesses lies in returning to our natural diet and lifestyle as described in chapter five. I also make mention of how to recover from sports related and overuse injuries, much of which I've learned from personal experience as a distance runner.

Returning to our natural diet and lifestyle as a way to recover from injury and illness in broad terms is a relatively simple concept, but one that I've put some of my own unique spins on and is worth exploring in more depth for anyone who is serious about reclaiming their health or avoiding disease. I sincerely hope this guide helps you or someone you care about discover the right path back to a healthy and happy life.

> "Believe nothing that depends only on the authority of your masters or of priests. After investigation, believe that which you yourself have tested and found reasonable, and which is for your good and that of others."
>
> *- Shakyamuni Buddha*

---

## ***Introduction and Disclaimer***

As you may have noticed, there is no Ph.D., M.D., or N.D. next to my name on the cover of this book. Though college educated, I am not a doctor, nutritionist, or a physician. What I've attempted to offer here is a model of human health based on studying I've done on my own and on listening to my body carefully for many years. Unfortunately, despite the legions of extremely educated individuals in society today who are working diligently to understand and cure disease, millions of people still suffer with fatigue and chronic illness and have no clear solutions to their health problems. This guide is my small contribution to that ongoing search for answers.

I hope the ideas herein offer fresh insight at the least and at best provide the answers you need to reclaim your complete physical and emotional health. My intention is not to claim this is the one and only way to heal, but rather that it's the way I believe makes the most sense based on my own experience and research. It is true that each person is unique and people have their own beliefs and ideologies and respond differently to different things. However, I hope the information in this guide can be of benefit to the majority of people suffering from chronic illness.

Parts of this guide may seem a little technical and at times may read like a text book. The irony is that (and I'll be the first to admit this) the process of recovering our health is actually not that complicated, but it's taken an in-depth look at how the human body evolved and functions to really prove, at least to myself, how the simple tenets of healing actually work their magic. I hope the reader comes to understand more specifically how our return to health depends on the interplay between hunger, food ingredients, and food preparation. Also remember that the first four chapters are directed more towards those with upper digestive weakness and fatigue. The ideas presented first then tie in to a more all-inclusive strategy for managing and overcoming chronic illness in general.

This book is directed towards those who are in a serious rut and are willing to stretch their minds a little to find a way out, and to muster the necessary discipline to succeed. For those who may fit in that category but who have little patience with science, I encourage you to focus your energies only on the parts of this guide that explain the role of acid in the body, the difference between "Active" and "Passive" digestion, and the diet and keys to food preparation.

To the more scientifically minded reader, and even individuals involved in fields of nutritional or biological research, I hope that some of the ideas I put forth might lead into new avenues of research that would increase our understanding of the link between food, lifestyle, and health. Since much of this work has grown out of what I've discovered by listening to my own body, the model for the cause and cure of chronic illness could benefit from deeper scientific validation of the reactions I've observed in my own body and heard of occurring in others with similar conditions. If such research nullifies, validates or in any way explains the theories I've put forth, or leads to a deeper understanding of the connection between diet, lifestyle, and chronic illness, the potential to help humanity's struggle with diseases of all kinds would be significant.

Research focused on curing illness through diet and lifestyle changes will not likely result in huge profits for the medical or nutritional supplement industries, since people will realize that the answers to their health problems may in fact be quite simple and within their own control. The medical industry as it is today often does more harm than good, both in terms of its effect on people's personal health along with the financial well being of our economy due to the vast expenses and inefficiencies involved. Pure scientific research, however, is not concerned with profitability; pure research has always been driven by the innate human desire to discover truth. In that spirit, I place my hope for the undertaking of any research inspired by this guide, and the funding thereof by foundations and sources interested in discovering the true nature of health and disease.

# 1

## *Dreams Deferred...*

*My background and philosophy on health*

While a sophomore at Vassar College in 1999 I came down with a stomach virus that for the most part ran its course in about five days. I'd run my body down over the past year and a half, maintaining a very unhealthy vegetarian diet (knowing virtually nothing about nutrition), running between 8 and 10 miles a day as part of the cross country team regimen and usually partying and drinking Friday nights before intense five mile races on Saturday mornings. I was a strong endurance athlete, but I treated my body like I was indestructible. I learned that I wasn't.

The stomach virus I contracted was probably nothing too uncommon (I remember there was something going around at the time), but because my defenses were weak, it hit me hard and had lasting effects. My first reaction soon after was to see a doctor who prescribed broad spectrum antibiotics in case I had some sort of stubborn bacterial infection...to no avail. The digestive and fatigue issues I developed could not be diagnosed by any allopathic or naturopathic doctor or specialist I saw. To this day, there has never been anything really "wrong" with me from a strictly medical perspective. The best anyone could do was to suggest I might have *Chronic Fatigue Syndrome*, or CFS. A *syndrome* is a set of symptoms with no established cause or cure. It's a medical professional's way of saying "we've seen this kind of thing before and named it, but we don't really know what causes it."

The next several years of my life were spent picking up where doctors, naturopaths, and healers of all kinds left off. I was determined to discover what was going on in my own body and committed to a quick and full recovery. I spent much of the first year nearly bedridden, using any windows of energy to run and exercise and finish school, convinced that soon I would reclaim my health and set records in cross country and perhaps triathlon later on.

Having graduated with a self designed major in *ethnobotany* (the study of how indigenous people use plants for medicine, food, and other purposes) which drew heavily on the disciplines of biology, chemistry and anthropology, I inadvertently laid a foundation for understanding the biology of the human body. As my search for answers deepened, I began to acknowledge there was nothing random or inconsequential about any bodily function, down to the behavior of every cell. That behavior could all be explained by looking at where we came from and how we got here through the process of evolution.

I read books on health and chronic illnesses including CFS, scoured the internet day and night (learning in the process that you can find almost anything you want to find on the net...as well as its opposite), experimented with different diets, supplements, fasts, and nearly every purported "cure" for whatever my latest theory was for the cause of my fatigue. I fully investigated yeast overgrowth, parasites, gallbladder/liver stagnation, bacterial infection, you name it. I studied healing systems of different cultures including India and China, as well as those of indigenous societies from various parts of the world.

Everything I targeted, I went at full bore. If it was yeast, I cut down on fermentable sugars and starches, eliminated fungi and yeast related foods from my diet to minimize immune cross reactions, tried antifungals of all kinds along with *probiotics* (beneficial bacteria) and so forth. I tried gallbladder cleanses, broad spectrum antibiotics, antiviral, antibacterial, and antiparasitic herbs and supplements of all kinds. I fasted multiple times including juice and water only fasts – once for five days on water alone. Fasting seemed to offer a temporary reprieve, but nothing worked in a lasting way.

I had a sonogram to check for gallstones and blood tests to check for bacteria and infection of any kind, all of which were negative. At one point I also had an endoscopy with a biopsy of my stomach that revealed only gastritis, which the doctor dismissed as a "common occurrence" and nothing to really worry about. I sent for tests for *Leaky Gut Syndrome* and a complete diagnostic stool analysis from Great Smokies Diagnostic Laboratory which revealed that indeed my stomach was "leaky," or more porous than normal, since a type of sugar that normally doesn't pass through the upper digestive system passed through mine after ingesting it and showed up soon afterwards in my urine. The increased porosity was attributed to inflammation (which could be brought about by anything from an infection to too much coffee or alcohol).

On a less pleasant topic, healthy people's stools are loaded with bacteria (up to 50% dry weight) which are themselves predominantly healthy and referred to as *probiotics* (meaning "for life"). These bacteria ferment fiber and help break down undigested carbohydrates in the colon, providing a significant source of energy for our bodies while producing vitamins, antiviral and antibacterial short chain fatty acids (SCFAs) and a host of other immune enhancing and anti-inflammatory compounds. They also help free up minerals and other nutrients for absorption into the body.

I had virtually none of these "friendly flora." This wasn't too surprising given all of the antibacterial, antiviral and antifungal supplements, herbs, spices, and medications I had taken to that point. It's also likely that my initial stomach virus back in 1999 had wiped out (due to extreme diarrhea as well as antibiotics I had taken) a lot of intestinal flora to begin with, which may have triggered the cascade of chronic infection and stomach inflammation.

The only other thing that showed up in the battery of tests I had gone through over the first couple of years following my stomach virus in college was a slightly elevated white blood cell count. Indicative, the doctor told me, of a very low level infection or tissue trauma of some kind, though no specific bacteria, virus, or parasite was ever identified.

Every bit of information I could get I held on to like gold. Every indisputable fact I could gather I used to build a foundation for my own understanding. If no one else could figure this out, I would. Every reaction to every meal, snack, or drink I consumed I researched and documented to decipher the mystery of my fatigue. I continually mulled over my symptoms, documenting reactions to meals, snacks and activities up to three or four days prior – all in an effort to hunt down a cause and pinpoint a cure. Mostly it was a feeling of utter stagnation; a full body malaise that took over very rapidly following food or drink, and remained for hours until my body processed it and rebalanced itself...usually only to be thrown off again with the next snack, drink or meal.

Over time, I started piecing together foods and activities that seemed to help, or "worked," and discarding things that didn't. My symptoms showed up within seconds or minutes of what I ate or drank, often leaving me bedridden for hours until they subsided. The ineffectiveness of the "*Candida Diet*" and the fact that symptoms would hit quickly and hard even after eating non-carbohydrate foods made me rule out yeast as a cause. Within a few months to a year I completely abandoned faith in pharmaceutical medications. No pill was going to cure me and I acknowledged that putting isolated, synthesized compounds into my body was not a natural, healthy thing to do.

Disheartened with medicine, I turned to herbs and supplements. I spent over two thousand dollars on various botanicals with most purporting to be the next magic cure-all (as explained within shiny tri-fold pamphlets filled with the shocking results of double-blind studies and testimonials from people on the brink of death now bounding through meadows with more energy than they ever dreamed of) with no luck. I lost faith in supplements and herbs, and the expense that went with them. Furthermore, if I came across a tempting supplement or herb, I would simply figure out its natural origin which was almost always found in some herb or spice I could obtain locally, and I just tried adding whatever that was to my diet. For probiotics, I turned to raw fermented and cultured foods. I figured it would be cheaper, more natural and more effective that way anyhow.

I remember talking to the boyfriend of a friend of mine, a doctor in his 50s or so, about four years after I contracted my stomach virus and was deep in my search for answers. We started talking, and he hinted that he could probably help me. After talking a little longer, he surmised that the problem was probably related to yeast and suggested I make an appointment to see him. I mentioned I had read about and tried the *Candida* diet and he started shifting uncomfortably a bit in his seat. Genuinely interested in the possibility that he might have something unique to offer though, I explained that I had tried nystatin and diflucan (two powerful prescription antifungals), as well as a host of natural antifungals followed by probiotics, and cut out sugars and fungi related foods that might have cross reactions with my immune system. He literally cut me off in mid sentence, saying, "You may know some things but you don't have the background in biochemistry and molecular biology to know what's really going on." We were sitting in the kitchen, my friend preparing a meal, and it was a very awkward moment. I was a house painter at the time, and obviously he was threatened by my knowledge of what he considered his intellectual territory. For the rest of the evening we avoided discussing health issues. I never made an appointment to see him.

    While some doctors truly love what they do and are instrumental in helping people overcome their health issues or avoid disease, I also think many doctors (at least the ones I've met and heard of) have become disheartened with their occupations, especially in the treatment of chronic illness. As the engines of modern health care, doctors are entrenched in an industry that is financially dependent on disease and strongly influenced by corporate profit. Pharmaceutical companies don't make their money from healthy people; they profit from the sick. It's not really in the interest of the modern healthcare industry (which employs a full 8% of the US workforce) to cure, but rather to treat indefinitely. Side effects of drugs are often handled with yet more drugs. It's an endless cascade that can leave a person dependent on medicines and at worst results in more extreme health problems or even death.

General practitioners and specialists are also now faced with "know-it-all" patients (admittedly including myself) who have spent days, weeks or years self-diagnosing with the help of the internet. The information revolution has been a thorn in the side of many medical practitioners who have worked hard and paid a high price to be in a position of intellectual authority over their patients, and they resent challenges to this authority (granted, often with good reason). The negative and defensive reactions I received from doctors the few times I tried to tactfully steer them clear of what I knew to be dead end paths made me realize I'd run my course with allopathic medicine.

In the evolution of my understanding of health and the human body, I went quickly from searching for a "magic bullet" – a pill I could get from doctors that would cure my symptoms – to approaching the search for answers and ultimately a cure from a more intuitive and holistic approach. The essence of that approach has been this: that all people ultimately have the *potential* to be healthy. For the most part, we're not born into this world with bodies that are destined to be sick. That would run counter to every reason that we're still here as a species. The genetic design of our bodies has evolved over hundreds of millions of years through natural selection back to the beginning of life itself; our ancestors survived the often extreme conditions of their environment and reproduced while those with less well-suited DNA (or bad luck, granted) did not. Our ancestors' DNA is our DNA. What's changed, and changed dramatically in the past few hundred years (a blink of the eye in the span of human evolution) is what we eat and how we live.

The human body is incredibly balanced, resilient, and adaptable, but we evolved to thrive in the context of the natural world; dependent on a wholesome diet and a physically active lifestyle. When pills and medications failed to heal, my search for answers began to shift from the *microscopic* to the *macroscopic* (and the one within the context of the other). To heal completely would be inevitable if one were to simply return to the context in which their body was meant to be in. Bones heal, muscles mend, infections are defeated, balance is restored. The human body tends toward health as water tends to flow downhill, so long as we adhere to our natural diet and lifestyle.

So what exactly is the Natural Diet and Lifestyle (or NDL)? One of my fundamental assumptions was that whatever made me consistently feel good, and could realistically be found in the natural diet and lifestyle of our ancestors, was indeed part of it. Whatever didn't make me feel good, or could never be found in the natural diet of our ancestors (like, say, refined flour or high fructose corn syrup), was indeed *not* part of it.

Anthropological studies of indigenous peoples around the world in the late 19th and early 20th centuries reveal diets that were entirely devoid of processed foods while the health of these individuals was robust, even given the highly unhygienic conditions they lived in. Chronic ailments like diabetes, arthritis, osteoporosis and obesity were virtually nonexistent. However, when European explorers infiltrated these societies and imposed their refined diet (white bread taking the place of tubers and so forth), the health of the indigenes quickly deteriorated.

To figure out what constituted the natural healing diet, I constantly tested different foods and ingredients to see what worked and what didn't. If I ate something that made me feel good, I would go back and see how that potentially fit in to the natural human diet. Through this process of "hypothesize and check, observe and hypothesize," I gradually pieced together the answers. Like a marble dropped down the side of a bowl, rolling towards the center then up the other side, then back down and up the opposite side, in time settling in the exact middle...what made sense in theory and worked in practice (and vice versa) became, to me, part of the Natural Diet and Lifestyle.

An example of the "hypothesize and check" pattern I followed was to test what initially made theoretical sense: the raw food diet. For a while I was convinced that only raw foods composed what early humans ate as their natural diet, since no other animal (including our close relatives the great apes) eats cooked food. I surmised that a raw food diet, therefore, would cure my problems. But after a few months on a raw food diet and constantly feeling weak and fatigued, the marble rolled up the other side of the bowl and lost momentum. I had to rethink how natural "all raw" actually was, especially given the inordinate amount of time, preparation and ingredients necessary to make meals that were usually not too satisfying.

Back at the drawing board (so to speak) I imagined the relative simplicity of a caveman throwing a hunted or trapped animal on a fire, turning it a few times, then eating it and feeling immensely satisfied and strong. Compared to gathering and soaking nuts, making nut "milk" and nut "cheeses," cutting up and dehydrating fruits and vegetables and making elaborate dishes...the raw food diet just didn't add up. Especially since after all that work and planning, my body still cried out for a juicy grilled burger, cooked starches, fried bacon, roasted chicken or baked pizza now and then.

To cook, people needed to be able to create and control fire. For cooked food to be part of the natural context of our DNA, it needed to have been going on for a significant period of time and had to have been a factor in our natural selection as a species. We know that *Homo erectus* migrated out of Africa about 1 million years ago, and for that migration to take place across Eurasia and into the colder climes our ancestors needed to be able to create and control fire. There isn't definitive evidence of exactly when our ancestors first harnessed fire (findings of fire "pits" in Kenya in the 1980's puts those man-made fires at 1.6 million years old.),[1] but scholars widely agree that beginning about 400,000 years ago controlled fire was widespread. Modern humans (*Homo sapiens*) came into existence about 250,000 years ago. Keep in mind also that natural selection is influenced both by duration and intensity. Though hundreds of thousands of years may not be extremely long in the big picture of evolution, the intensity with which our ancestors used fire, especially with our migration into colder parts of the world, was extreme. Cooked food was not a luxury, it was a *necessity*.

Four factors eventually forced me to recognize that cooked food is part of the natural human diet: 1) anthropological evidence of controlled fires by our ancient ancestors; 2) the necessity of controlled fires in the process of human migration around the world; 3) my own and many others' undeniable craving for cooked food especially meat and starch, and the uniquely satisfying, empowering, and healing effect it has on our bodies, and 4) the use of cooking in every major society and culture around the globe and throughout recorded history. Obviously this is not to say that all our food must be cooked, but only to say that *some* cooked food is a healthy part of our natural diet.

In this guide I describe similar explorations of biological pathways within the human body that have arisen through evolution and explain what I consider to be the cause and cure of most, if not all chronic

---

[1] http://www.dichotomistic.com/mind_readings_fire.html.

diseases. I unite some fundamental concepts from modern science with ancient medical and healing philosophies from different areas of the world under the same umbrella.

# 2

## *Answers...*

*An attempt at a unification theory*

I'm convinced the final triggers of all chronic diseases boil down to the following: excess acid and toxins in the body, insufficient oxygen/nutrients, or a combination of both. The root causes of these triggers are poor diet, toxic indulgences and lack of exercise and/or rest. Between the root causes and final triggers lies the realm of chronic illness; from infections to chronic inflammation to Diabetes, Crohn's disease, CFS and Cancer. Behavioral and mental illness also often originate and/or are perpetuated by chemical and physical imbalances in the body, though of course emotional trauma can trigger these imbalances as well.

In Traditional Chinese Medicine (TCM) which originated several thousand years ago, health is understood to be determined by the flow of life force, or Qi, within a person. This Qi in turn results from the two opposing forces of the universe; yin and yang. When one's Qi slows or stagnates due to an imbalance of yin and yang, a person becomes ill.

Practitioners of TCM view everything in the universe as a reflection of its opposite, down to matter itself. Male and female, day and night, hot and cold, good and bad, positive and negative...all are expressions of yin and yang which are illustrated in the following familiar symbol:

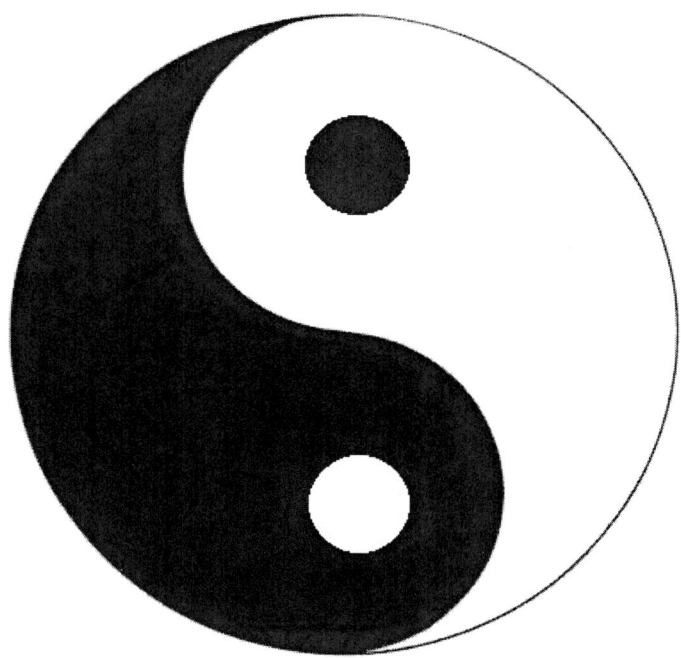

*Chinese symbol of Yin and Yang*

Yang represents the masculine, bright, hot, acidic, and imposing force in the universe, while the yin force is feminine, dark, alkaline, cool, and receptive.

Modern chemistry also describes matter as being composed of particles with opposite forces: protons and electrons. A third particle, called the neutron, exerts neither a positive nor negative force, but adds to the size and weight of the elements. Chemical reactions in nature as well as in the body are caused by the opposite charges of protons and electrons, which attract each other with an equal and opposite force. Protons are at the center (or nucleus) of atoms, while electrons orbit the nucleus and can be stripped away from the nucleus by positive charges of other nearby atoms or molecules.

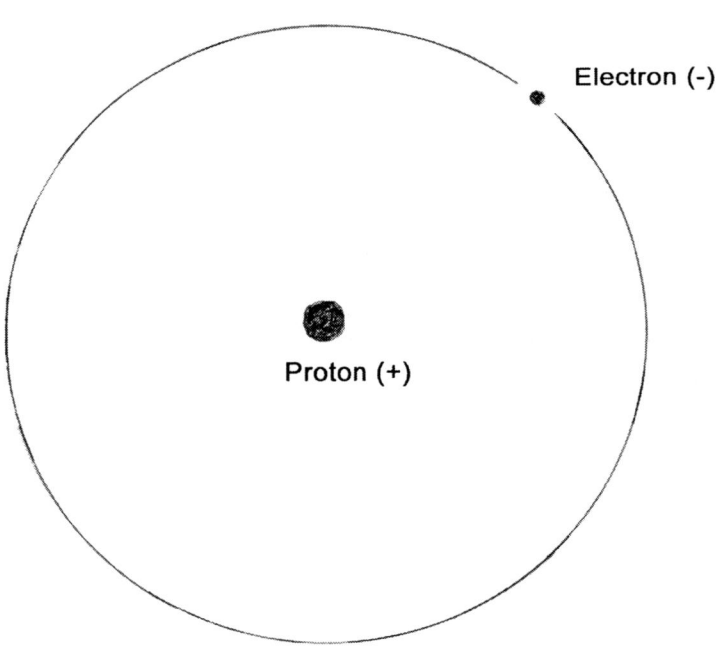

*Hydrogen atom (the smallest element with only a single proton and a single electron)*

Notice the similarity between the ancient Chinese view of the universe and human health, and the actual building blocks of matter discovered through modern chemistry. Every atom and therefore all the matter composing our bodies consist of opposites; protons and electrons. As it turns out, the balance between protons and electrons is one of the most important aspects of health in the modern perspective as well.

A proton without an electron orbiting it to balance out its charge is an acid. Molecules (composed of atoms) from which protons can dissociate in solution are also acids. An example would be hydrochloric acid (HCl), or stomach acid. Acids, which "steal" electrons from other elements or molecules to balance out their charge, are therefore also known as *proton donors*. On the other hand, an element or molecule with an excess of electrons in proportion to its protons is an alkaline substance.

*Acidity and alkalinity, or yin and yang in TCM, are fundamental to the balance of human health.*

The body is essentially an acid production factory, since acid is a byproduct of energy metabolism in every cell. In addition our stomachs produce and maintain a strong concentration of acid in order to kill harmful microbes and digest food. Yet despite the constant production of acid in our bodies, human blood must remain slightly alkaline to bind oxygen and carry out all the functions of supporting the life of our cells. Our cells must also remain slightly alkaline and so our bodies are in a constant state of producing, sequestering, and getting rid of acid before it builds up and causes disease or kills us.

To reiterate (because this is important), *an acid is any element or compound that has an excess of protons and therefore is a proton donor.* These protons are free to travel (in a solution, such as water) and "steal" electrons from other elements or compounds since protons and electrons are opposites and attract each other to balance out their charges.

The scale that measures the concentration of an acid is called the pH scale, which stands for "potential Hydrogen." The scale is logarithmic, which means between each consecutive whole number on the scale there is a ten-fold difference in acidic concentration (between three consecutive numbers like 1 and 3 there is a 100 fold difference, between four consecutive numbers is 1,000 fold, etc). The scale goes from pH 0 to pH 14, where pH 0 is most acidic, pH 7 (in the exact middle of the scale ) is exactly neutral, being neither acidic nor alkaline (such as pure water), and pH 14 is the most alkaline, or basic.

**STRONG ACID** -------------------------------------------------- → **STRONG BASE**

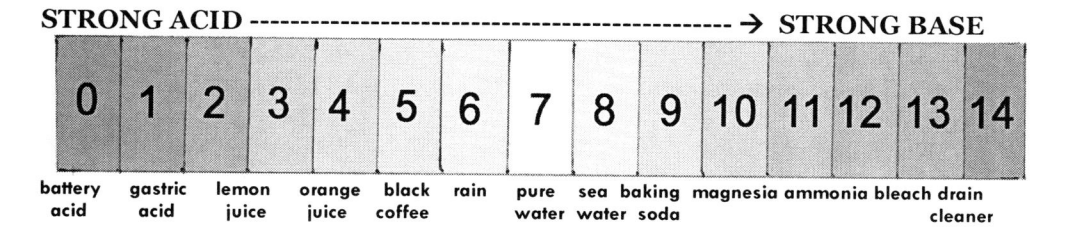

| 0 | 1 | 2 | 3 | 4 | 5 | 6 | 7 | 8 | 9 | 10 | 11 | 12 | 13 | 14 |
|---|---|---|---|---|---|---|---|---|---|----|----|----|----|----|
| battery acid | gastric acid | lemon juice | orange juice | black coffee | rain | pure water | sea water | baking soda | magnesia | ammonia | bleach | | drain cleaner | |

*The pH scale*

**Essential Concept**:

The pH of human blood is slightly alkaline, and restricted to the narrow range of pH 7.35 to 7.45. The body will do everything possible to keep blood in this pH range. If it falls out of this range, blood cells lose their ability to bind oxygen and death will follow within seconds.

When cells burn fat, protein or carbohydrates for energy, they produce acid as a byproduct. This acid is pumped into the blood and exhaled through the lungs as carbon dioxide. Acid is also "buffered," or absorbed in the blood by proteins and amino acids which act as temporary sponges, either being expelled through the urine, feces, or releasing the acid gradually to be dispelled as carbon dioxide.

When the body stagnates (or the flow of Qi is impeded) due to lack of exercise, poor circulation, an acidic diet, or blockages due to inflammation or infection, acid can build up. An acidic diet is one in which the acid produced from cells metabolizing the calories of the food outweighs the alkalizing nutrients of the food. Therefore, most "whole" foods are alkaline and processed foods are acidic. This build up of acid can be localized or more generally systemic, but in either case the drop in pH of blood (that is, the increase in acid concentration) lowers the oxygen content of the blood and infection, inflammation, and even diseases such as cancer can take hold and spread.

Though our blood and tissues are constantly producing and getting rid of acid, there is one place that acid is produced and sequestered in large quantities: our stomachs. If the stomach lining that separates that acid from our blood ever breaks down, a cascade of health issues will ensue, as I will soon explain.

SYNOPSIS OF HEALTHY DIGESTION

In healthy people, the stomach retains a very low pH from acid secreted from the wall of the stomach. This "resting" pH is around pH 2.0, or slightly stronger than fresh squeezed lemon juice. Stomach acid is important for the following reasons:

1. Strong acid destroys harmful bacteria, viruses, fungi, and parasites
2. Strong acid begins the process of breaking down protein and enables proper functioning of the protein digesting enzyme *pepsin*.

3. Strong acid keeps upper digestion moving; food in the stomach passes from the stomach into the duodenum (a 12 inch long tube that forms the first part of the small intestine; see diagram on following page) more readily when the acidity is strong enough. Without strong enough acid, the "nozzle" separating the stomach from the duodenum (called the pyloric sphincter) closes and food stagnates in the stomach and flows back into the esophagus.

The stomach senses the concentration of acid by proteins in the lower stomach wall (just as surface proteins on our tongues let us know that lemon juice is acidic). When the pH rises above 3.5 (a guesstimate on my part), the proteins signal the stomach to essentially halt digestion until more acid is secreted to bring the pH back into its effective range.

As the acidic food contents of the stomach, called *chyme,* pass into the duodenum, the acidity is neutralized by extremely alkaline bile which is manufactured in the liver from red blood cells, salts and fatty acids and stored up in a sack under the liver called the *gallbladder.* Bile, along with other enzymes and alkaline bicarbonate produced in the pancreas, neutralize acid and further break down fats, proteins and carbohydrates as they pass into the small intestine. When food reaches the large intestine, beneficial bacteria (*probiotics*) ferment any remaining undigested carbohydrates (including fiber) and release nutrients that are absorbed into the body before final expulsion of the waste. In healthy individuals, there are *more bacteria in the colon than cells in the body*, and the vast majority of these are beneficial.

That's digestion, in a nutshell. The diagram on the following page illustrates the digestive system for reference:

## Human Digestive System

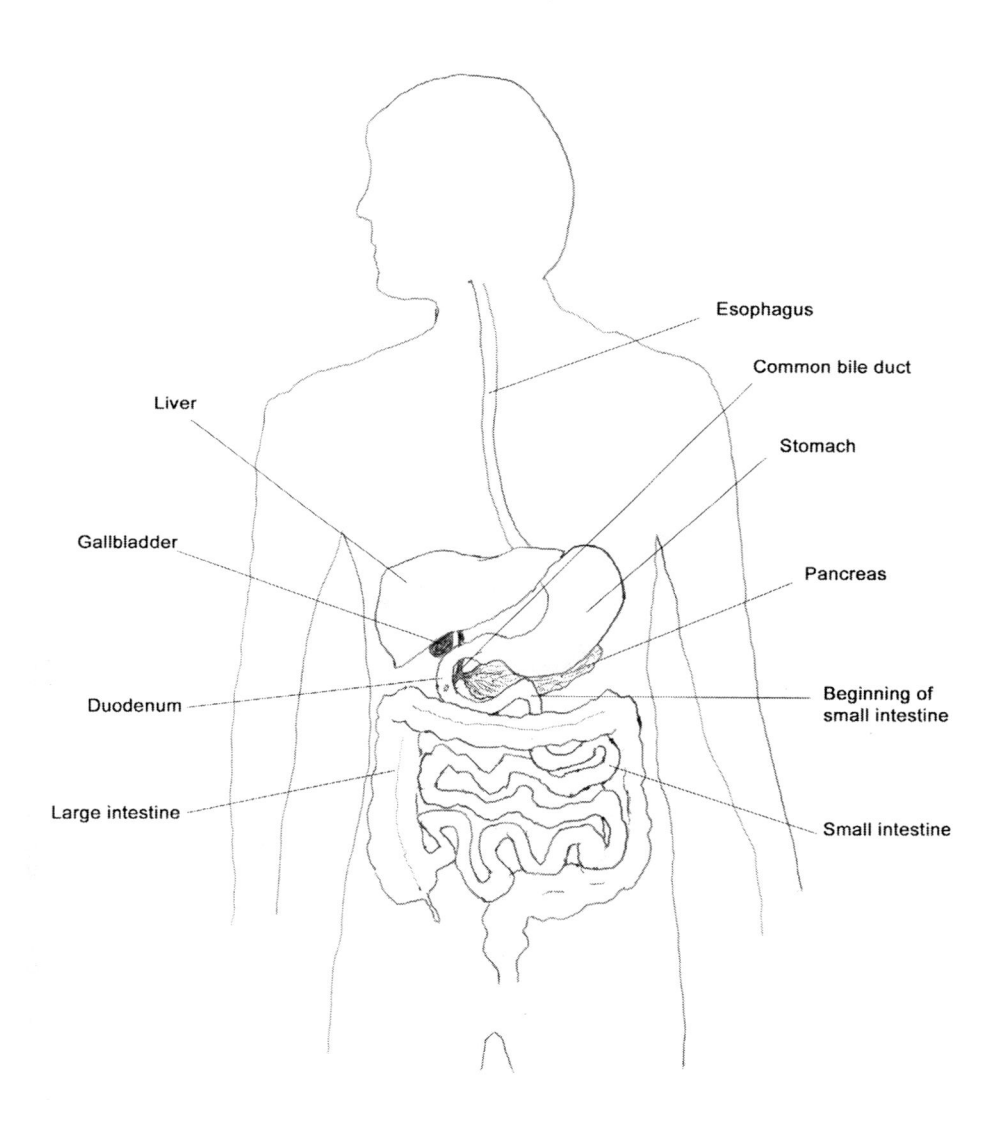

*Note the stomach, duodenum, liver, gallbladder, pancreas, small intestine and large intestine (colon)*

The digestive system utilizes extreme degrees of acidity and alkalinity while protecting the blood from these fluids and selectively absorbing nutrients and expelling toxins across the digestive lining.

A healthy person maintains a healthy digestive lining from the stomach wall down into the duodenum, small intestine and large intestine. The large intestine is home to an abundance of probiotics which primarily thrive on carbohydrates and fibers that our own digestive enzymes can't break down. Our digestive health and overall well-being are profoundly dependent on these beneficial bacteria which produce important nutrients and short chain fatty acids (such as *acetic* and *propionic* acid) while inhibiting harmful microorganisms from taking hold in our digestive system.

Because the digestive system is a primary barrier that all harmful bacteria, viruses, yeast, and parasites must penetrate in order to eventually infect the body, over half of the body's immune system is located along the digestive tract. The digestive system is just one example of a *semi-permeable membrane* within our bodies. Nearly every "compartment" of our body is contained within a semi-permeable membrane, from our cells to our digestive organs to our entire body within our skin. We are living sponges, selectively taking in what's around us, processing it, and secreting the waste back into our environments in a highly regulated and controlled manner on which our health depends.

In a healthy person, the semi-permeable membranes of our cells, organs, and digestive system are strong and do their job effectively. Our stomachs are intensely acidic, bile and pancreatic juices are intensely alkaline, our blood is slightly alkaline, and the flow of fluids across these membranes is tightly controlled. In my view, the compartmentalization of digestion parallels the separation of charges across membranes at a cellular level, creating the electrical potential and life-force in our bodies. This separation of opposites across membranes - the polarization of yin and yang within our bodies - is a central characterization of a healthy individual. It creates the dance of energy and life within us.

On the following page is a simplified diagram of a healthy individual, illustrating how these opposing charges are separate and strong within the body.

# Healthy Individual

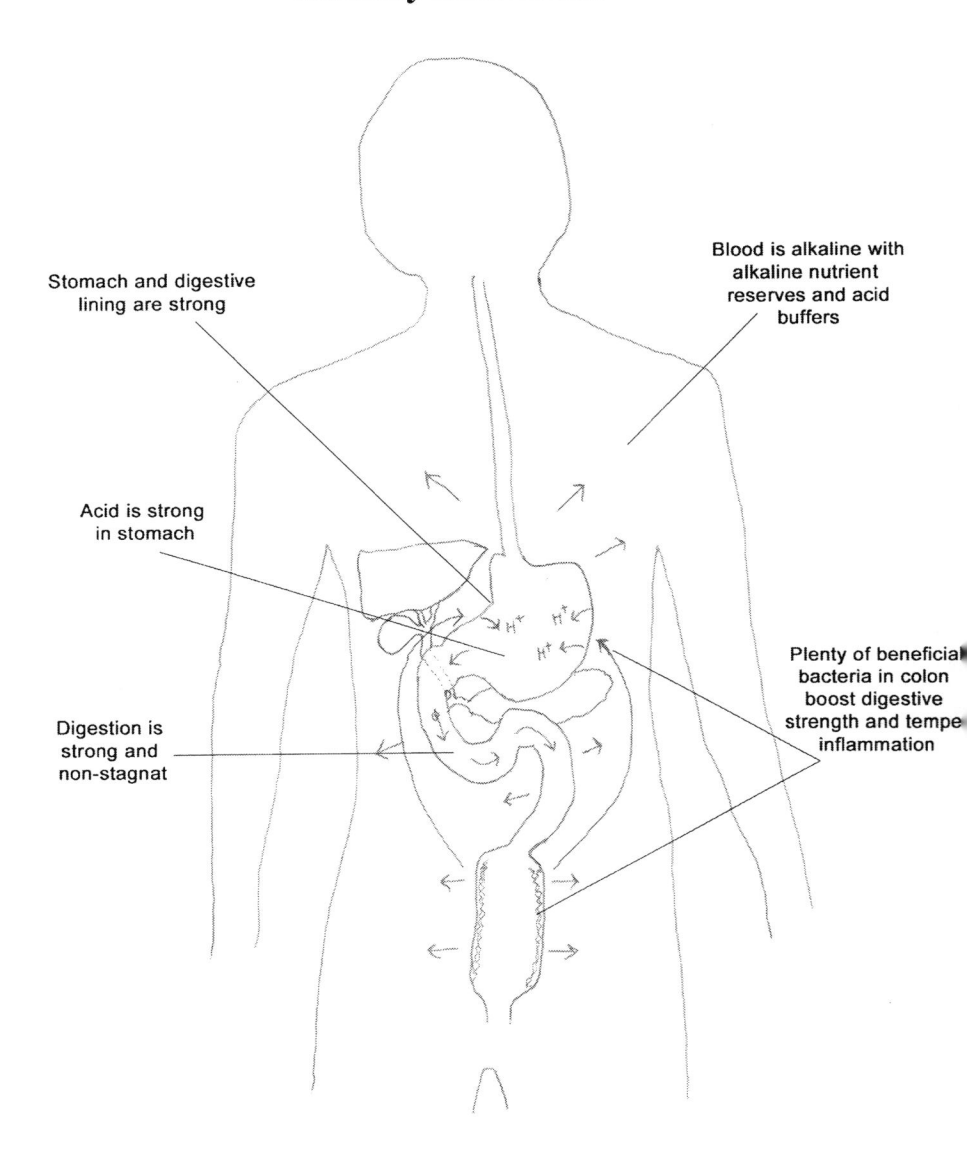

**Stomach and digestive lining are strong**

**Blood is alkaline with alkaline nutrient reserves and acid buffers**

**Acid is strong in stomach**

**Digestion is strong and non-stagnat**

**Plenty of beneficial bacteria in colon boost digestive strength and tempe inflammation**

*Healthy person with strong Yin-Yang life-force*
*(Small and large intestine are simplified, H+ represents hydrogen acid ions)*

# COMPROMISED DIGESTION AND ACID-BLOOD CROSSOVER: AN EXPLANATION FOR CHRONIC FATIGUE

*Synopsis: A viral infection triggers inflammation of the stomach, making the stomach lining more porous. Acid produced in the stomach lining then leaks back across the porous lining into the blood, aggravating inflammation and disturbing the sensitive pH of the blood, causing symptoms of CFS.*

The beginning of my illness was marked by a week-long stomach virus, which I mentioned in the introduction. After that I was not the same. My digestion was weak, I was constantly fatigued, and I developed strong intolerances to drinks and foods that were milky or creamy (not necessarily dairy, but anything of a milky or creamy texture), sweet, pasty (such as soft bananas or overcooked starch), or bland. More details later about the food "triggers" I developed, but suffice to say my digestion was somehow deeply compromised after that week long stomach virus.

Also as mentioned in the introduction, the only positive results that came of a multitude of doctor visits and dozens of tests including an upper gastrointestinal endoscopy (where the physician looks into your stomach with a camera and take a biopsy) was the following:

1. Slightly elevated white blood cell count indicating a prolonged low level infection
2. Presence of gastritis, or inflamed stomach lining
3. "Leaky gut" (due to inflamed stomach lining)

4. Lack of healthy intestinal flora

A few years after I had my stomach flu, I became severely ill and tested positive for *mononucleosis* after driving from Florida to Maine on little sleep and fast food along the way. I realized that the symptoms of mono were very similar to those of my regular fatigue symptoms, and after researching mono more in depth, I found that one of the common symptoms between mono and what I had going on was gastritis.

Having gained much knowledge of nutrition and how to deal with my regular fatigue symptoms, I was able to get rid of my mono in a relatively short period of three weeks by controlling my diet and getting plenty of fresh air (for many people mono lasts months or upwards of a year). Ironically, it was the contracting of mononucleosis and realizing the similarities of symptoms between my regular fatigue and digestive problems and those of mono that led to the theory that fatigue was caused by the "leaking" of stomach acid across the porous and inflamed stomach lining into the blood. Recall the pH scale and the immense difference in acidity between stomach acid and blood, and the fact that our blood must always remain in a very narrow, slightly alkaline range to bind oxygen. Since there was no definitive explanation for what exactly caused the fatigue associated with mono, I figured powerful stomach acid and an inflamed stomach were to blame.

I realized acid was a major player in my illness since symptoms would rapidly dissipate sometimes after vomiting. Because of my digestive weakness, food would sit in my stomach and cause the miserable feeling of fatigue and stagnation that's hard to describe unless you've felt it. It's like being poisoned while food in the stomach sits high up, refusing to be digested. As time goes on the feeling gets worse; fatigue and irritability set in, digestion shuts down completely until after awhile the *only* relief is vomiting. I remember at times only acid would come up, but I would immediately feel much better and so I began to link acid to my symptoms. Once my stomach was empty and resting my body would come back into balance and the fatigue would dissipate (but usually only until I ate or drank something again, until I began to figure out how and what to eat).

The times I did vomit were never induced by anything but my own digestive weakness and absolute physical fatigue, stagnation, and malaise. I've been told by people who have had eating disorders that perhaps I too had an eating disorder, which was frustrating in that it insinuated a psychological aspect to the reaction. Mine was a digestive problem; food stagnated in my stomach and caused a debilitating physical reaction. How to describe it? I felt like a plant wilting in the sun while being poisoned at the same time. My pulse would skyrocket while my body and head felt like lead. Nothing I could eat or drink would make it better (I tried that in the early years; it only made things worse).

I eventually pieced the puzzle together and came out with this explanation: the stomach flu I contracted in college was a virus (like the mononucleosis virus) which took hold due to my severely rundown body and poor diet. The infection caused severe diarrhea which, along with the antibiotics I took, wiped out much of the friendly flora of my lower GI tract. The stomach virus was eventually brought under control by my immune system but perhaps never fully eradicated. In either case, inflammation of my upper stomach (gastritis) became chronic and caused the stomach lining to become more porous, or "leaky." This was often accompanied by a sore throat. As a result stomach acid production fell (acid-producing cells called "parietal" cells are located in the mid and upper portion of the stomach where the inflammation was), and the acid that was being produced and secreted from the stomach wall in turn aggravated the inflammation and leaked back into my blood. The test from Great Smokies Diagnostic Laboratories showed that larger sugar molecules could pass through my inflamed stomach so I surmised that surely the much smaller acid ions could as well (in healthy individuals with a healthy stomach, normally the only substance that can penetrate the stomach lining and pass into blood is alcohol). I concluded the leaking of acid across the inflamed stomach lining disrupted the highly sensitive blood pH and caused the full-body malaise I was experiencing.

# Stomach Acid-Blood Crossover

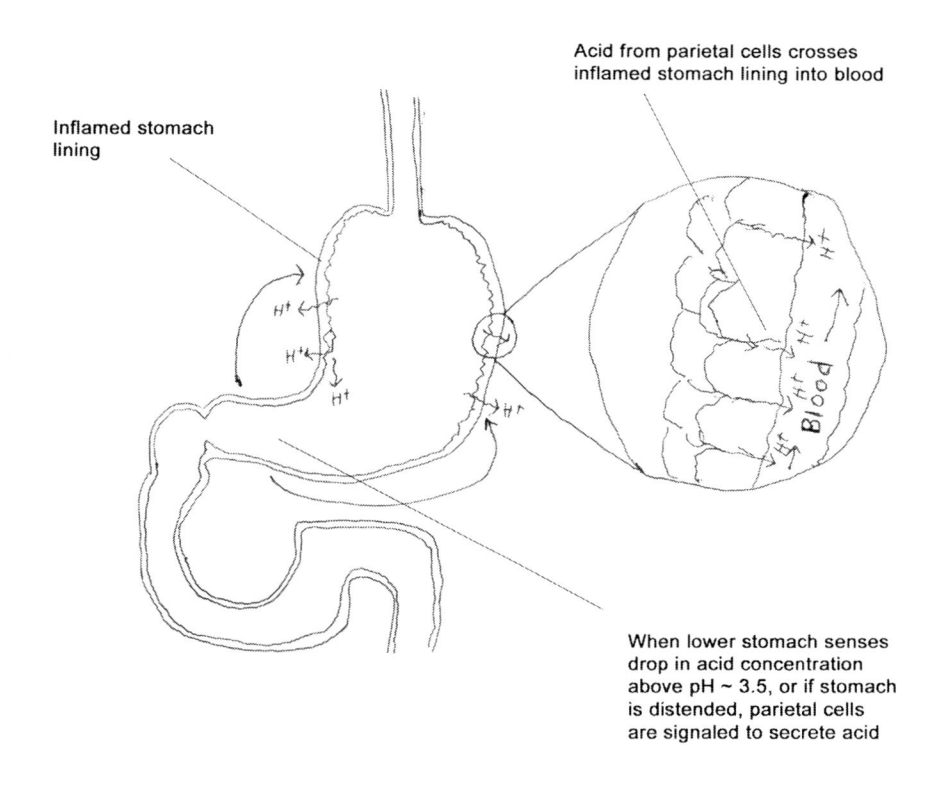

*Inflamed and porous stomach with acid-blood crossover*

Initially I decided to try simply neutralizing my stomach acid with milk and antacids, but this caused symptoms to return in force. I realized that it wasn't so much the acid already in my stomach that was the problem; it was the acid being produced and secreted from the stomach wall that was immediately seeping into my blood. Since the stomach only increases acid secretion in response to distention (stretching) or a drop in acid concentration due to food or liquids, milk and antacids only worsened the situation and caused "rebound acid secretion." It also seemed that when the stomach was stretched with food, or *distended,* the porosity of the inflamed tissue would also increase (like needle holes in a balloon would increase in size when the balloon is filled with water.) Indeed, symptoms were bad and would last the longest on a full stomach.

Even with compromised acid production due to gastritis, the concentration of stomach acid when it's being secreted from the stomach wall (that is, as it's exiting the canals of the stomach lining) is pH 0.8, while blood pH must remain exactly 7.35 – 7.45. That means stomach acid, as it's being secreted, is about *3 million times more acidic than arterial blood*, so even the smallest amount crossing the inflamed gut lining at that point would have a huge impact on our overall health and energy. However, as acid gathers in the stomach it is diluted to pH 1 – 3…still extremely acidic!

Remember that proteins on the stomach wall sense the acidity of the stomach contents, and when the acidity is not strong enough (when pH rises above 3 or 3.5) the stomach must slow down and secrete more acid to regain the necessary concentration for safe and efficient digestion. With gastritis, acid secretion is compromised due to the inflamed stomach lining and the upper digestive process easily stagnates.

The cascade continues with food not being broken down and efficiently absorbed, which keeps the body from obtaining the supply of nutrients it needs for energy, healing, and effective immunity, and the cycle of chronic illness maintains itself. Inflammation also gets out of control due to the lack of healthy intestinal bacteria that help regulate and temper inflammation. From the perspective of a healthy person living as compartmentalization of opposites, CFS results from a breakdown of a major barrier allowing yin stomach acid and yang blood to merge.

# Individual with Gastritis-Induced Chronic Fatigue

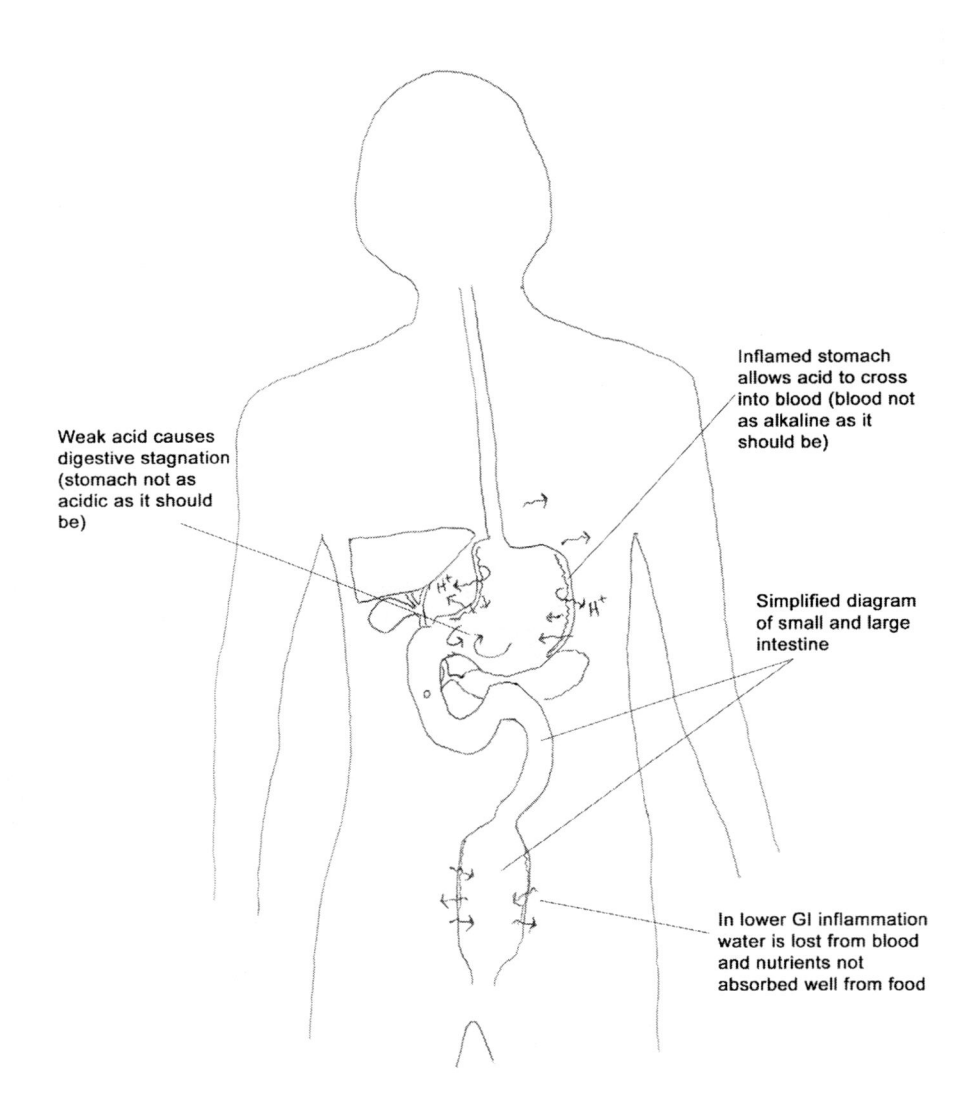

Inflamed stomach allows acid to cross into blood (blood not as alkaline as it should be)

Weak acid causes digestive stagnation (stomach not as acidic as it should be)

Simplified diagram of small and large intestine

In lower GI inflammation water is lost from blood and nutrients not absorbed well from food

*Sick person with break-down of yin-yang life-force
(Small and large intestine are simplified)*

Over time, I came to realize that certain foods were especially effective at triggering symptoms while other foods seemed to have the opposite effect. After eating them (when hungry) I felt my digestion was virtually back to normal. There was no stagnation and I felt grounded and strong. But again these effects only occurred on a relatively empty stomach and when I was hungry. Eating anything when I wasn't hungry would always result in fatigue and digestive stagnation.

**Essential Concept**:

Because of the extreme difference in how I felt after eating certain foods at certain times, I hypothesized that the human body has evolved two different pathways of digestion. I refer to these two pathways as "*Active Digestion*" (AD) and "*Passive Digestion*" (PD).

After years of experimenting and documenting my body's reaction to food I learned exactly what foods had positive effects (triggering Active Digestion) and what foods and drinks triggered my symptoms (through Passive Digestion). The essential difference between the two is that in Active Digestion, eating cooked animal protein-fat (APF) when hungry and, to a lesser extent, raw leafy greens signal the stomach to stop secreting acid and send the food down to the next chamber, the *duodenum*, where powerful digestive fluids from the gallbladder and pancreas aggressively break down food. AD is not dependent on acidic breakdown of food from the stomach. Passive

Digestion, on the other hand, occurs in the absence of AD triggers or hunger; food sits in the stomach and slowly enters the duodenum passively, as long as it has been sterilized by the strong acid of the stomach.

In Passive Digestion, unless food in the stomach is sufficiently acidic, the pyloric sphincter will close and the duodenum will not allow the chyme to enter (possibly as a defense mechanism against pathogenic organisms). My theory is that AD overrides the acidity of the stomach since other powerful digestive fluids are set in motion that will break everything down in the duodenum anyway.

I also discovered that I could tolerate some of the PD "trigger" foods if I ate the AD "empowering" foods first, or if I waited until I was extremely hungry at which point I could tolerate a moderate amount of almost any kind of food. Gradually, I developed a method of breaking the cycle of digestive weakness and chronic illness based on understanding the interplay between food, digestion, and hunger, along with exercise and rest.

What really excited me was that the entire interplay fit perfectly with what would have been our Natural Diet and Lifestyle. As active hunter-gatherers, the spoils of the hunt would constitute a meal in itself after the meat was prepared and cooked. By the time we ate, our digestion would be primed and hunger would be strong, just as the smell of cooking bacon or hamburgers seems to trigger a primal craving unlike any plant-based food does.

Before we get too involved in what foods stimulate Active Digestion and how, a little background in nutrition will come in handy. By understanding the basic properties of food and its interplay with digestion we can better control what we eat and ultimately how we feel.

# 3

## *A Crash Course in Nutrition...*

*Humans need the full spectrum of macro and micro nutrients*

The Natural Diet and Lifestyle is eating and living in a way that is harmonious with the "intentions" of our design. That is, giving our bodies what we need to be strong physically and emotionally while eliminating extreme substances that which the inherent balance that our health depends on.

To better understand what the natural human diet and lifestyle consists of, we must begin with a basic understanding of food and nutrition as well as the digestive processes required to break down and absorb the food we eat.

Everything we eat can be divided into two basic categories which are termed *Macronutrients* and *Micronutrients*.

Macronutrients are nutrients we need in relatively large amounts to provide us with the calories we burn on a daily basis. The four macronutrients are:

1. **Protein (4 calories per gram):** (made up of amino acids, of which there are 23 total; 8 essential and 15 non-essential. If the body gets the 8 essential, it can manufacture the 15 non-essential from them.) A few important functions of proteins are: to act as

acid buffers or "sponges" in the blood, to rebuild muscle and body tissue, to act as an energy source.

2. **Fat (9 calories per gram):** (or fatty acids, of which there are short chain, medium chain, and long chain.) A few of the many functions of fatty acids: compose hormones which regulate body functions including inflammation, used as energy source, compose cell membranes.

3. **Carbohydrates (4 calories per gram):** (sugar, sugar molecules linked together to form starch, and sugar molecules linked in different ways to form soluble fiber and insoluble fiber.) A few functions of carbohydrates: they are the preferred energy source of the body and probiotic bacteria, fiber cleanses the digestive system, binds to cholesterol in bile and helps detoxify the body.

4. **Water (0 calories):** A few functions: cleanses, cools, and keeps things moving in the body. All chemical processes in the body take place in the medium of water.

In terms of calories, the average adult person who is moderately active burns about 2,000 to 3,000 calories per day, and the ideal ratio of calories from macro nutrients which maintain and fuel the body is in the range of 10 -15% protein, 30-40% fat, and 45-60% carbohydrate. Keep in mind fat is over twice as calorically dense as protein or carbohydrate, so the 30-40% refers to calories from fat and not a physical proportion.

*Micronutrients*, as the name implies, are the nutrients we need in smaller amounts but are still absolutely necessary in maintaining our health, and include:

1. **Vitamins** (fat soluble vitamins A, D, E, and K, and water soluble vitamins B complex and C) – the "spark plugs" of metabolism and many chemical reactions in the body.
2. **Minerals** (including those we need in large [macro] quantities sodium, potassium, calcium, magnesium, phosphorous, iron, and those we need in trace amounts such as iron, chromium, iodine, fluoride, and many more) – the building blocks of everything we're made of. Minerals are essential in everything, including maintaining the pH balance of our bodies.
3. **Phytonutrients** (all other nutrients in plants that may confer health benefits for their anti-inflammatory or antioxidant properties)
4. **Probiotics** (beneficial bacteria in raw and fermented foods that colonize the large intestine and boost health)

Minerals are perhaps the most significant aspect of modern nutrition that people overlook in their diets. Most processed foods are either stripped of their minerals or supplemented with excess minerals (such as sodium or calcium) which can even lead to the stripping of other minerals from our bodies in the process of secreting the one mineral that was added in unnaturally excessive amounts. This risk is not present for the most part in whole foods, which have a natural mineral balance.

Certain minerals such as calcium have been hyped up beyond their true relevance by industries with an incentive to sell their foods or products which happen to be rich in that mineral. Calcium, however, is no more important than any other mineral in the diet, and while the recommended daily intake (RDI) for calcium is around 1000 milligrams, the RDI for potassium is over three times that – 3,500 milligrams. Potassium has the effect of balancing out sodium on the outside and inside of cell membranes, which directly affects blood pressure. Processed foods such as canned soups, preserved meats, or fast foods can easily tip the balance of the minimal sodium-potassium ratio within the body and lead to all kinds of health problems. Keep in mind also that the potassium RDI of 3,500 milligrams is the minimum; a natural whole foods diet along the lines of what our ancestors ate was likely much higher in potassium, and much, much lower in sodium. One more note on potassium (since it's the mineral we need most abundantly and is often the most lacking in processed foods): nearly all fruits and vegetables are abundant in it. Grains are quite low in potassium, but rich in other minerals so combining breakfast grains with fruits or whole fruit juices, or adding fruits and vegetables to all meals will help ensure an adequate daily potassium intake.

All nutrients can be either lacking in our diets (leading to malnutrition) or sometimes consumed to excess at which point they become toxic. Even water when consumed in excess can be toxic and even deadly. In human nutrition, everything is best when in balance.

The main problem with modern food production is the stripping of micronutrients from foods and the raising of plant foods in mineral depleted (and often toxic) soils. Meat, eggs and dairy from animals that have been raised in industrial farming operations with nutrient depleted, toxic feed and in cramped, filthy environments pass their imbalances and toxins on to us. We are what we eat. A steak from a cow that was raised in an open pasture is much healthier in every way (including higher in anti-inflammatory omega-3 fatty acids which are found in algae and leafy greens) than a steak from a cow that was raised on quick-growth diet of grain and antibiotics and injected with growth hormones.

Carbohydrates are themselves often stripped of fiber and refined to white flour which is a nutritional ghost of its whole grain origin. White table sugar and high fructose corn syrup are both nutritionally empty sources of quick calories. Fats too are often processed and stripped from the whole food sources they're derived from.

The end result of consuming these processed foods is that the body metabolizes the calories and produces acid and toxins as bi-products which degrade the body over time without retaining the micronutrients (or beneficial bacteria) that are present in whole foods. These micronutrients are necessary for the body to rebuild itself and fight off illness and disease, and the health effects of a processed foods diet are cumulative. Small inconvenient health issues will turn into full blown chronic ailments over time if such a diet is maintained.

The difference in how we feel and look after a few months on a natural, whole foods diet with organic, free range and wild animal and plant sources of food compared to how we look and feel after a few months on denatured, processed, refined, industrial food sources is the difference between night and day. In addition, by adhering to a natural and whole foods diet we can avoid contributing to the immeasurable suffering of animals bred, raised and slaughtered in industrial operations.

# 4

# *Active Digestion (AD) and Passive Digestion (PD)*

*Synopsis: I've come up with the term "Passive Digestion" to describe what takes place when the stomach senses a drop in acid concentration (from too much food, sugary liquids, acid dilution, etc), triggering rebound acid secretion which penetrates the inflamed stomach wall into the blood. "Active Digestion" is my description of the more powerful and energy-expensive digestive process that takes place in the duodenum (between the stomach and small intestine), during which time stomach acid is turned off. Active Digestion is responsible for the aggressive breakdown of macronutrients. Fatigue symptoms can be avoided by eating meals that trigger AD instead of PD.*

Most food and drinks have the effect of "buffering" or absorbing and diluting acid in our stomachs and raising the pH. When the proteins on our stomach wall detect this rise in pH above about 3.5, they signal the stomach to secrete more acid and get the pH back down in order to ensure neutralization of harmful microbes and to help begin breaking down food. It's during this time of stomach acid secretion that people with gastritis-induced CFS experience the symptoms of acid-blood crossover.

The pH-detecting proteins in the stomach wall sense a rise in pH from several main causes including:

1. The buffering of stomach acid due to sheer quantity of food.
2. The buffering of stomach acid due to the acid-absorbing quality of food or drink. For example milk is an extremely effective acid

buffer and neutralizes acid quickly, causing the stomach to secrete more acid in response.

3. Food and drinks that coat the stomach wall and themselves are not very acidic, including milk and most sauces, marinades and dressings that have acidity above pH 3.5. This also occurs when eating extremely soft or pasty starches such as overcooked grains, potatoes or thick soups or sauces. All these things can coat the stomach and trigger rebound stomach acid secretion.

4. Acid-detecting proteins on the stomach wall are tricked into sensing a decrease in acid concentration in the stomach by dissolved sugar. Sugar of any kind in solution actually competes with acid for binding sites to proteins. When sugar from a sweet drink or a sweet snack coats the stomach wall, acid does not, and the perceived pH rises immediately. Just as lemon juice tastes less acidic when sweetened with sugar, the stomach senses less acidity when sugar is coating the stomach. Digestion grinds to a halt until the stomach can secrete acid and restore the necessary pH.

As previously mentioned (on p. 39), I refer to this process of the stomach responding to its perceived level of acidity by secreting more acid simply as "Passive Digestion," or PD. The symptoms of Passive Digestion are magnified when the stomach is both distended with food (increasing its porosity like a stretched balloon) and the inflammation is aggravated with acid secretion or harsh substances such as alcohol or coffee.

Active Digestion (AD), on the other hand, is triggered in response to strong hunger and the uniquely rich nutrient source of animal protein and fat (APF). I learned of it by feeling it and researching the digestive processes in response to different nutrients. Whenever I was hungry for and made APF a significant part of my meals, I felt much better; grounded, strong, and back to normal. APF is most effective when protein and fat are in combination. Butter is a mild AD stimulant (lacking protein), and extra lean meats are also mild (lacking fat), but meats that are tender and a little fatty are most effective.

The Active Digestion pathway makes sense from an evolutionary perspective as well. As humans evolved as hunter-gatherers, the successful catching of fish and hunting of wild animals was the single greatest possible addition to the menu. Nothing else filled, grounded, and empowered us in one fell swoop as did the meat of wild birds, fish or game. When we were lucky enough to catch such a meal, we better have had the digestive wherewithal to break it down and absorb it efficiently. However, Active Digestion is a somewhat energy-expensive process and can only happen when the body is hungry and ready for APF.

Indigenous cultures the world over prize meat above other foods. Constantly exposed to pathogenic microorganisms and parasites, indigenous societies that live as close to the natural world as our ancient ancestors did have relied on meat to boost their health and immunity and to empower them physically in ways that plant based foods never could. One reason is that, because of its protein density, the acid buffering potential of meat far outweighs any plant source. In recognizing this, the hunting and killing of animals for food has been a practice steeped in spiritual gratitude and the recognition of human-animal kinship all the way back to prehistoric times.

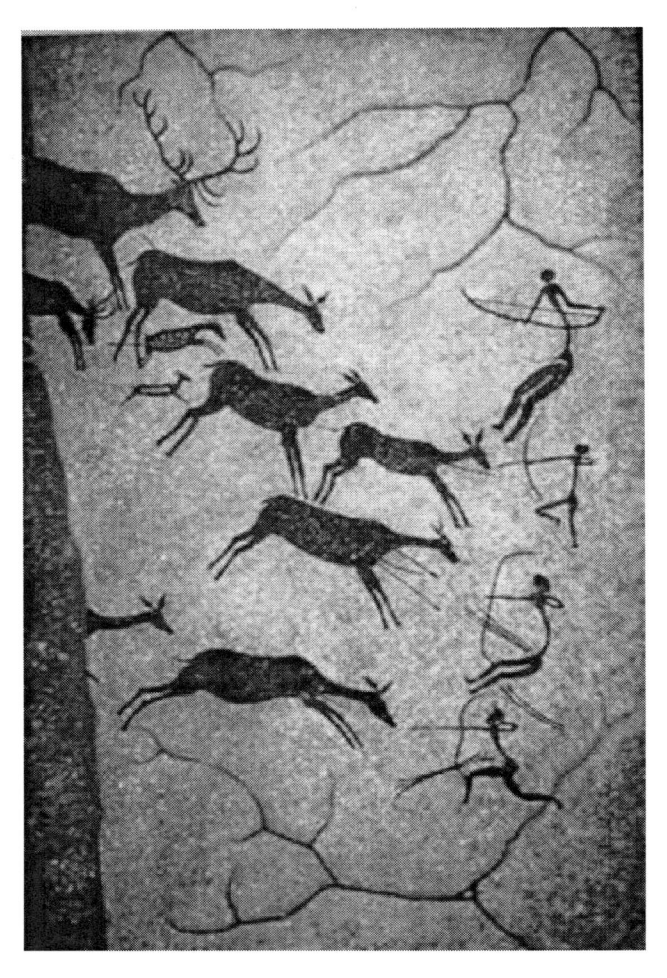

*Prehistoric cave painting from Lascaux, France (17,000 BCE) depicting the hunt*

Today, animals remain an important part of the human diet the world over. Our cravings for bacon, eggs, grilled chicken, steak or fish are undeniable, though many choose to maintain vegetarian or vegan diets, or various other diets for any number of reasons. The fact remains that we benefit greatly from organic, free range, and/or wild APF as part of our natural diet, and the AD pathway exists due to recognition of this important nutrient source.

When you're hungry for and eat APF on an empty stomach, the protein-cholesterol matrix is detected in the duodenum and Active Digestion is triggered.  Cholesterol is one type of fat produced only in the animal kingdom and it is integral to stimulating AD.  To be detected by cells in the duodenum, APF has to be bio-available; not bound up in a sauce or starch matrix, and warm enough (i.e., cooked/melted) for the fat and protein molecules to easily separate and be absorbed.

In AD, the hormones *secretin*, *glucagon* and *cholecystokinin* (CCK) are released when APF is detected in the duodenum.  These hormones inhibit gastric acid secretion.  At the same time, the protein digesting enzyme *pepsin* is released in the stomach along with mucus, which coats and protects the inflamed stomach wall.

As stomach acid is turned off, the liver and gallbladder gear up to release bile that will mix with food in the duodenum, along with pancreatic enzymes.  These fluids are the essence of Active Digestion.  They are powerful and filled with protein, fat and carbohydrate digesting enzymes and work relentlessly to break down animal protein and fat (APF).

Once Active digestion is triggered, the inhibition of stomach acid and secretion of mucus that coats the stomach wall keeps acid from aggravating the inflamed gut wall and crossing into our blood.  The APF is being subjected to much more powerful digestive fluids than acid in the digestive cauldron of the duodenum. However, the AD pathway requires significant amounts of energy and only occurs in the presence of strong hunger. Hunger is the primal signal that our digestive system is in fact ready to get to work. In those with chronic illness due to compromised digestion, it's important to only eat meals when hungry. Eating without hunger or over-eating will cause food to stagnate and symptoms will flare up in full force.

APF triggers Active Digestion but other nutrients help enable it, especially minerals. This is why a balanced diet rich in fruits, vegetables, and leafy greens is essential. Without sufficient minerals from these foods, the body and digestive system weakens, becoming more acidic overall, and causing inflammation to flare up. Those with digestive disorders especially need a constant supply of mineral rich foods in their diet especially, since healthy intestinal flora that help facilitate mineral absorption are usually lacking.

If one is craving nutrients or a sugar boost but hunger is not present or digestion is weak, then only the most basic nutrient rich and low calorie foods are tolerable, watered down fruit juices or juicy fruits, brothy (not thick) vegetable soups with lemon juice, simple salads, bland and low calorie vegetables lightly steamed and lightly dressed with lemon juice and salt, for example. These foods will be absorbed passively without much digestive exertion, and will build back the power of digestion and the body overall.

## Active Digestion and Raw Leafy Greens...

Besides APF, raw leafy greens stimulate Active Digestion as well while also alkalizing the body. Based on what I feel happens in my own body, it seems that when you chew up and swallow raw greens, the juices coat the stomach wall and stimulate bile flow and AD. In addition, leafy greens are one of nature's most powerful anti-inflammatories; they are truly nature's medicine. In addition, raw greens picked from rich, organic soils are good sources of beneficial bacteria (along with other vegetables and fruits grown in such soils). I'm not sure how leafy greens do it, but I never fail to feel it. This is another area where more research might provide answers.

Given the importance of hunger with regard to APF and Active Digestion, greens are an effective addition to the diet when your digestion feels weak or inflamed and you want to restore your digestive strength.

## Understanding Surface Interactions...

*Synopsis: Food and drink do not affect us until they interact with our digestive lining. They're not "part" of us until they pass through our digestive lining and into our blood and cells. Also, to temper the effects of acid secretion, acid must be cut off where it's produced in the parietal cells of the stomach lining where it can immediately penetrate the blood. Buffering acid that has already been secreted is not helpful.*

When considering the effect of food and liquid on health, you need to remember that there is no effect until the food that is chewed and swallowed contacts the surface of the gastrointestinal tract itself. A lump of rat poison in the stomach is completely harmless so long as it floats within the contents of the stomach and is not absorbed into the body. Technically, the digestive tract is like our skin; it separates what is outside of us from what is inside of us. Digestion, and therefore health, is only influenced by interaction between what we ingest and the surface of our digestive lining. This concept is powerful because it explains how certain foods and fluids may have a different and sometimes opposite impact from what we expect.

For example, I assert that acid is the cause of the symptoms of fatigue and malaise, and secretion from the stomach wall aggravates inflammation of the stomach wall itself. In my case, the solution seemed simple at first; neutralize the acid with milk or antacids. Yet every time I did this the symptoms were immediately much worse. After much thought, I realized what was going on. By buffering what little acid that was in my stomach, I triggered a rebound reaction in which my stomach began secreting acid to bring the pH back down to normal levels. As that happened, acid secretion in the gastric pith (the canals from which acid is released out into the stomach) immediately aggravated the inflamed tissue and penetrated into my blood before even exiting the stomach lining.

Another example of a surface interaction is the case of APF. As discussed, APF has the ability to trigger active digestion, but only when it comes in contact with the surface cells of the lining of the duodenum. This surface interaction cannot happen if APF is "bound up" in a starch matrix, or if APF is eaten *after* other foods, and is therefore sitting on top of foods that have already triggered PD. So we can't just say "Oh, meat is the answer. Even though I just ate a bowl of ice cream and feel bad, if I eat a steak now I'll feel better." Such eating patterns would never have been part of the natural diet and lifestyle.

## Keys to Food Preparation; the Importance of Consistency and Texture in Triggering AD:

*Example: boiled soggy dark chicken meat affects digestion differently from grilled chicken breast with spices; though both are chicken. Mashed potatoes have a different effect than French fries, and so forth.*

As you now know, bland and sweet foods that coat our stomachs trigger Passive Digestion and cause the symptoms of CFS. This applies not only to foods that are "soupy" before eaten, but foods that become liquid in the mouth by mixing with saliva before being swallowed, such as chocolate or candy. Fluffy, flour based foods such as pancakes or cake turn back into batter consistency in our mouths, which then coats the stomach and triggers PD. The same goes for thick soups of any kind, such as split pea soup or even soups with thick broths that have been cooked too long.

Overcooked, soggy vegetables can be problematic too. Vegetables are best when lightly steamed or cooked just to the point of being fork-tender. Foods that are served in thick, "gunky" sauces (for example, most Chinese take-out dishes) or salads with an excess of thick dressing are equally troublesome. Soft and sweet fruits such as ripe bananas or melons turn into purees before swallowed and can likewise trigger PD. The only way to eat such things and avoid PD is to eat them when extremely hungry or after eating APF/greens (when hungry) that trigger AD first.

This is why nearly every meal seems to be troublesome to people with gastritis-induced CFS. It's not just *what* we eat that matters. It's also the consistency and texture of what we eat that influences upper digestion, along with the sauces and flavorings we use. By understanding how the texture of a food after chewing triggers symptoms, we can learn to prepare foods accordingly. For example, instead of pancakes, opt for well cooked crepes made from whole white wheat flour (yes, there is such a thing!) and milk. These are extremely nutritious, heavier, dryer, and chewier than pancakes and will remain semi-solid in the stomach instead coating and buffering the stomach which causes rebound acid secretion.

Eggs also are either tolerable or intolerable depending on how they're cooked. If wet and runny, they coat and are problematic. When overcooked, they're not recognizable as APF either since the yolk is solid. But cooked "medium-well" or poached, the whites become slightly solid but the yolks remain slightly runny, cholesterol/protein is detectable and AD is triggered.

Rice, oatmeal and other grains and starches can be troublesome if cooked too long, they can be overly soft and pasty, turning into a puree when chewed and swallowed. When cooked just enough or even "al dente," they don't turn into a puree when chewed and aren't nearly as aggravating, if at all.

Yogurt can have a similar effect as milk. After being swallowed, it coats and aggravates gastritis by triggering rebound acid secretion. However, small amounts are tolerable on a hungry and empty stomach, or if Active Digestion is set in motion first. Raw yogurt with active cultures of beneficial bacteria can be included in the diet in small amounts since it is a rich source of nutrients and probiotics.

Spaghetti with tomato sauce is another perfect example of a dish that can be subtly manipulated. When cooked and served with the sauce on top, the sauce tends to coat the stomach lining and aggravate gastritis. However, if you "cook the sauce in" to the pasta a bit or use just enough to coat the pasta you can avoid the problem. Served with organic meatballs that aren't soaked in the sauce, you've got APF that is detectable and not in a sauce matrix and therefore able to trigger AD, making it a meal that won't aggravate symptoms. Add a side salad of raw greens and you should feel even better.

### *AD vs PD: A Power Struggle...*

*Active Digestion cannot override Passive Digestion, but Passive Digestion can override Active Digestion*

Ok so you're hungry, you start off with some APF, a cheeseburger or grilled chicken breast perhaps, along with a small side salad. You're feeling good and can tell you're in an AD state. So what happens if you eat another plate of food on top of that or drink a glass of milk? Can stomach distention and acid buffers halt and overpower AD? Yes, they can. Perhaps not immediately, but if stomach acid is extremely buffered and the stomach is distended, PD will kick in naturally to help break down food and kill pathogenic microorganisms that might begin fermentation. Remember from an evolutionary perspective, the stomach is mostly a storage sack for big meals (food was never guaranteed so when it was available we had to eat as much as possible). If those meals went bad in our stomach, we'd be done for. Acid keeps that from happening.

On the other hand, if rebound acid secretion is stimulated from buffering food, liquids, or stomach distention, it is impossible to override Passive Digestion with Active Digestion at that point, so always eat your meat before your pudding!

Remember also that everything can be taken to excess. All things our bodies (and I would venture, our souls) need, when consumed in excess become toxic. This is especially true in the case of food when digestion is compromised. When APF exceeds digestive capacity, or when APF oils coat the stomach wall (affecting perceived stomach pH) instead of sinking to be detected in the duodenum, the stomach is easily sent into PD mode. Excessive oils such as in French fries or extremely greasy meats will not only be a caloric burden to a compromised digestive system, but will also tend to coat the stomach lining and trigger rebound acid and PD.

### *Active Digestion and Hunger...*

If you're hungry enough, even acid buffering foods and starches are tolerable despite gastritis and compromised upper digestion. One reason for this is when you're really hungry, the stomach is small and shrunken and the inflamed tissues are hardly exposed. Food won't sit in the stomach for long when we're really hungry, our body will move things along to absorb nutrients as quickly as possible. Therefore, AD is the default digestive pathway when we're very hungry.

One reason daily exercise is important is because it leads to hunger and stronger digestion. When really hungry, you feel that no matter what you eat, you'll digest it. Take advantage of these opportunities to eat exactly what you want, be it yogurt, cereal, fruit, etc. Once you satisfy the strong cravings, make sure your next meal is balanced so as not slip back into PD mode.

## Summary: Shifting the Digestive Burden from the Stomach through Active Digestion

The stomach is essentially programmed to secrete acid and remain acidic as it holds food that is to waiting to be digested. This is called Passive Digestion, and has evolved primarily as a way of sterilizing food in the stomach. Acid is produced and secreted via parietal cells in the upper part of the stomach where chronic gastritis is also present. The stomach is signaled to secrete acid when:

- It senses a rise in pH above 3.5, especially in the lower part near the duodenum due to buffers or dissolved sugars
- It is distended with food and/or liquid

The secretion of acid from the stomach in the presence of gastritis causes acid-blood crossover and the symptoms of fatigue. While the stomach tries to regain its proper pH, digestion stagnates and nutrient absorption is stalled, magnifying fatigue and symptoms.

To mitigate rebound acid secretion, it helps to acidify foods and drinks with fresh lemon juice or vinegar. The acidity of food in drinks is nowhere near as strong as acid secreted from parietal cells, and is not a risk in acid-blood crossover.

The stomach is signaled to STOP secreting acid when the acid concentration is sufficient (pH under 3.5) or if Active Digestion is triggered when:

- Stomach is empty and hunger is strong (i.e., after a long workout) – good opportunity for fruit, yogurt, cereal, whatever you're really craving, without side effects.
- Stomach is empty and cooked APF is eaten first.
- Raw leafy greens are included with meals.

Inflammation of the stomach flares up in response to certain aggravating substances, including:

- Tannins (bitter coffee, red wine, etc.)
- Alcohol

These are at best tolerable only on an empty stomach since their effects are much worse when the stomach is inflamed or distended. Cayenne pepper is a unique irritant that in small amounts stimulates mucus secretion and protects the lining of the gastrointestinal tract.

By including APF and/or raw leafy greens with meals when hungry, the digestive burden is shifted from the stomach to the duodenum, the "tube" that precedes the small intestine where alkaline bile and pancreatic enzymes mix with food from the stomach and break it down into absorbable nutrients. When Active Digestion is in motion, the stomach is signaled not to worry about secreting acid, but to "just pass it on down and we'll take it from here."

## Active Digestion

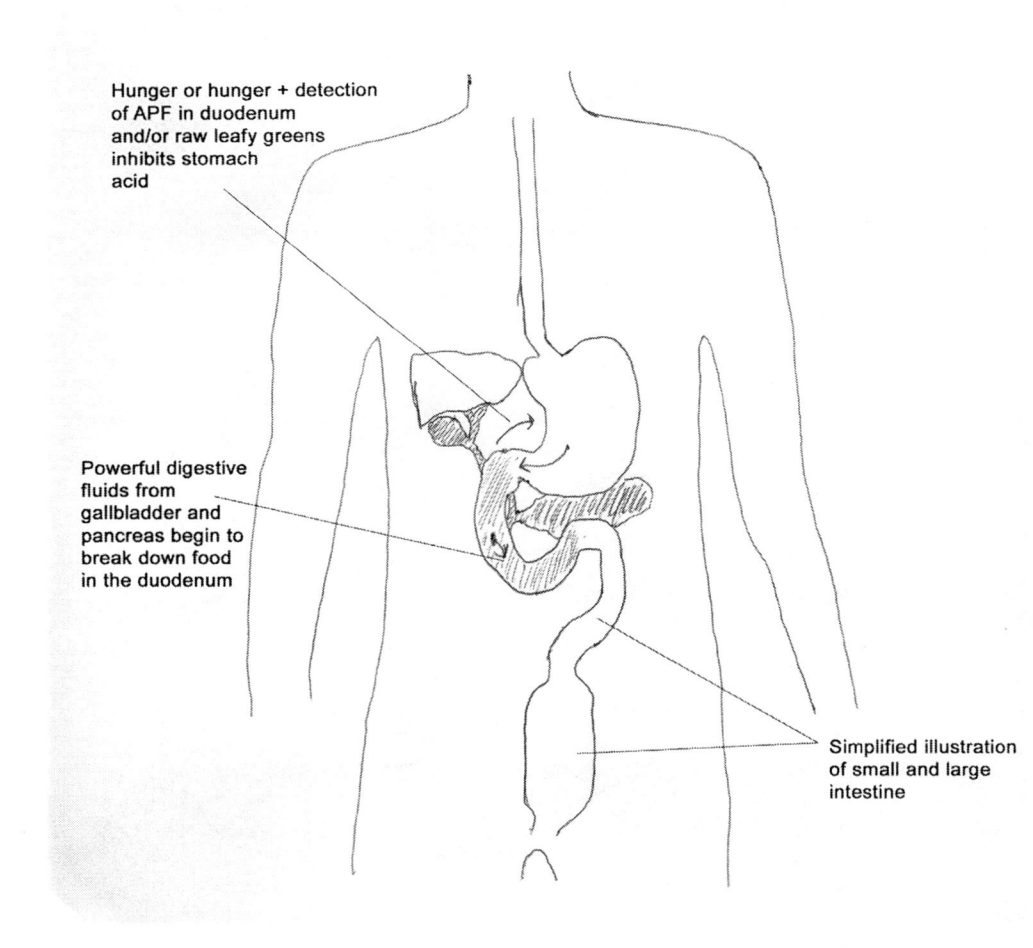

Hunger or hunger + detection of APF in duodenum and/or raw leafy greens inhibits stomach acid

Powerful digestive fluids from gallbladder and pancreas begin to break down food in the duodenum

Simplified illustration of small and large intestine

*AD occurs in the duodenum which is separated from the stomach by the pyloric sphincter (involved shaded areas include pancreas, gallbladder, and duodenum)*

Active Digestion is dependent on hunger and eating APF on a relatively empty stomach, since it is only stimulated when APF is detected in the duodenum. However, if APF is eaten within a thick soup, sauce, or starch matrix (or for example as a small hamburger inside a large bun or chicken deep-fried in too much batter), it won't be as detectable as if it were eaten alone and therefore would be less effective at triggering AD.

The same problem applies to eating raw greens within a starch matrix. For example, when the juices of raw greens are absorbed into bread or anything else, they aren't detected by the stomach wall and can't impart their healing properties. Likewise, cooked greens can't impart their bitter juices on upper digestion since cooking wilts and locks in the bitter elements of greens. The nutrients are then released slowly over the entire course of digestion; slowly imparting alkalizing minerals but not stimulating AD as raw greens do. I discovered this after failing to feel the immediate effect of cooked greens as opposed to raw leafy greens.

One final note about the role of APF in the diet: if you think of the digestive system as a set of muscles, then just like other muscles they require consistent "workouts" to be kept strong. All of the digestive organs and muscles that our body employs to break down APF need that stimulation in order to stay efficient and strong, which results in better overall digestion and health.

## 5

## *A 5-Part Approach to Recovering from CFS and Chronic Illness...*

*Synopsis: The three components of upper GI induced CFS, namely viral infection, acid secretion, and inflammation, cannot be cured with medications. The approach must be holistic, and encompass five equally important parts which are pertinent to overcoming illness in general: 1) Shifting the digestive burden from the stomach to the duodenum and lower GI tract; 2) Healing with balanced, alkalizing and anti-inflammatory meals that support friendly digestive flora; 3) Riding the circadian hunger cycles; 4) Reducing/eliminating aggravants, and 5) Maintaining a physically and mentally active lifestyle.*

If CFS is caused by acid in the stomach passing through a more porous, inflamed stomach lining into the blood due to a chronic low level viral infection, then it would seem sensible to simply turn off acid production with medications, target the viral infection with antivirals, target the inflammation with anti-inflammatories, or medicate all three at once, right?

Unfortunately, medications have harmful side effects and the natural functions of the body have reasons for existing. Before interrupting normal body processes with drugs, one should always look closely at why those bodily functions exist in the first place, as well as the side effects listed for the medication.

"Switching off" acid production with H2 blockers or proton pump inhibitors (PPIs) essentially eliminates a major component of digestion, which would contribute to upper gastrointestinal stagnation and fermentation. Further, blocking acid completely would inhibit the passive breakdown of food into absorbable minerals and nutrients (the protein digesting enzyme *pepsinogen* requires an acidic environment to activate), and possibly lead to fermentation of food by pathogenic bacteria, yeast, and parasites further down the digestive tract in the absence of AD.

    Research has indicated that absorption of vitamin B-12 depends on a compound that binds to it called *intrinsic factor* which is produced by the acid-secreting parietal cells of the stomach. Medications that block the secretion of acid by parietal cells also inhibit the secretion of intrinsic factor, over time leading to vitamin B-12 deficiency. These are just a few of the many vital roles of stomach acid which, if shut down completely, would potentially create more problems than it would solve.

    What about targeting the underlying viral infection with herbs, supplements, and/or drugs? The problem with that is, unlike bacteria, yeast, or parasites, there is no effective virus-killing drug out there. Viruses are the smallest and most ancient forms of life, and they burrow deep within our cells and target our very DNA. Antiviral medications amount to chemotherapy; they kill off our own cells (including healthy ones) along with viruses in hope that the virus dies before we do.

    The only way to effectively exterminate a virus is through the body's ancient and highly developed immune system and a natural process of cell suicide, called *apoptosis*. Armed with the nutrients and oxygen our immune systems need, and aided by the armies of probiotic bacteria and yeast that provide antiviral and anti-inflammatory substances, our bodies and immune systems are extremely effective at eliminating any sort of viral infection. Immune cells destroy foreign invaders by engulfing them and bombarding them with oxygen - literally tearing them apart! If there is one guiding principle to fighting off chronic disease it's that our bodies are smarter and better at it than our minds are. We just need to provide the nutrients and get out of the way.

Finally, what about breaking the cycle by targeting the inflammation? If we can get rid of stomach inflammation, won't that break the cycle of acid crossing over into the blood and allow the stomach to heal enable the immune system to get rid of the underlying virus?

Unfortunately, all anti-inflammatory medications including steroidal and non-steroidal anti-inflammatories (NSAIDs) have side effects on the stomach itself that actually aggravate inflammation. Anti-inflammatory medications weaken the stomach lining and can cause ulcers and even gastritis in people who previously didn't have it. Targeting inflammation with herbs and different natural supplements can be mildly effective but won't cure the problem alone. The powerful acid secreted by the stomach that constantly coats the inflamed stomach wall is too aggravating.

Given that we cannot simply turn off acid, kill the virus or get rid of the inflammation with medications, what, then, is the answer?

The answer is to do all three together at once in a natural way...by shifting the digestive burden from the stomach to the duodenum and lower digestive system and eating a natural diet that supports and alkalizes the body, decreases inflammation, brings back our healthy intestinal flora (which also decreases inflammation and boosts immunity), and gives us what we need to heal in a holistic way.

## PART 1: SHIFT THE DIGESTIVE BURDEN FROM PASSIVE DIGESTION (PD) TO ACTIVE DIGESTION (AD)

*Synopsis: By eating meals that stimulate AD, the stomach can rest and heal while food is broken down in the duodenum and lower digestion.*

As described in the previous chapter, we can avoid symptoms of CFS associated with stomach acid secretion by eating balanced meals with APF and raw greens and only eating when we're hungry. By shifting the digestive burden away from the stomach and building back the healthy flora in our colon, the stomach and digestive system as a whole will heal over time.

Also remember that dissolved sugar competes with acid for binding sites on pH detector proteins on the stomach wall, giving a "false impression" to the stomach that the acidity is not strong enough and consequently triggering Passive Digestion. Juices should be diluted to "just sweet enough" and increase their acidity in proportion to their sweetness, minimizing the PD trigger. In nature, most fruits are somewhat acidic and tart to begin with. However, others are quite sweet and not very acidic at all such as bananas, papayas and melons, in which case the solution is to eat them in combination with more acidic fruits or add lemon juice to them.

PART 2: HEALING WITH BALANCED MEALS

*Synopsis: Regular, balanced meals trigger AD and flush and cleanse the digestive system while providing the minerals and nutrients our bodies need. The fiber and bulk of balanced meals also helps remove toxins and restore healthy intestinal flora with the inclusion of raw, unpasteurized fermented foods.*

Balanced meals will satisfy both hunger and the body's nutritional needs in order to heal and avoid cravings that cause slip-ups. Not every meal and snack needs to be balanced in and of itself but at least one and preferably two meals a day should be balanced with organic APF, whole food starches, fruits/vegetables, dairy and raw leafy greens.

Balanced meals help in healing in several ways. First, they take advantage of hunger and Active Digestion to include starches and sometimes sweet fruits and juices that, on their own, would trigger PD. This makes it possible to satisfy the body's nutritional needs without triggering fatigue symptoms.

Second, balanced meals include good amounts of soluble and insoluble fiber and bulk which help clean the digestive system and remove stagnating acid from the stomach, cholesterol and toxins in bile that have been filtered from the blood through the liver. In addition, the bulk from vegetables, fruits, and whole grains gradually alkalizes the body and provides a food substrate for beneficial bacteria in the colon which are often missing or out of balance in people with digestive problems.

Finally, by including small amounts of raw fermented foods such as cheese, yogurt (not enough to trigger PD), unpasteurized sauerkraut, kimchee, or any other raw ferment with active cultures in meals, one can re-introduce probiotics to the digestive system. These colonies of beneficial flora in turn produce vitamins and short chain fatty acids in the colon which fight harmful bacteria and yeast, boost the immune system, decrease inflammation, heal the gut and maintain healthy digestion.

## PART 3: RIDING THE CIRCADIAN HUNGER CYCLES BACK TO HEALTH

*Synopsis: Our bodies go through several cycles of hunger every day. If one of these "hunger-windows" is missed, the body's metabolism slows along with its "house cleaning" (since food bulk is not available to remove toxins) and an opportunity to build and heal is missed. Strive for a regular meal regimen.*

If you're a person who tends to sleep in or skip breakfast you may not know it, but after 8 hours of not eating (sleeping) your stomach is empty and your body is hungry, though it's in fasting mode. This assumes that you have been eating three or four regular, balanced meals a day. However, this early hunger can pass unnoticed if we sleep through or simply ignore it and have a cup of coffee or two and a small sugary snack to hold us over until late morning or noon. Breakfast was aptly called "break-fast" because a good night sleep is essentially a mini fast.

For people afflicted with gastritis induced CFS, this period of early morning hunger represents a window of opportunity for healing. If not taken advantage of, it can become the opposite; a time when acid is secreted in the empty stomach, stagnates, and throws off our blood pH yet again. Ever wonder why sometimes you can get up in the very early morning a lot easier than you can if you sleep in and try to get up a little later? It's because our stomachs are ready for food and our bodies are ready to move, but we don't eat and instead remain stagnant. Our stomachs fill with acid and our cells release acid and metabolites into the bloodstream that have built up over hours and hours. This is why I believe oversleeping makes us drowsy and more exhausted than ever.

Although I'm not aware of it right away when I get out of bed early most mornings, within 15 or 20 minutes I'm suddenly ravenous. By eating a good sized balanced breakfast at this time I always get off to a good start. My metabolism gets that early boost and I'm hungry again by mid or late morning (as long as I'm somewhat active), and again by mid afternoon, and again by late evening. This is the natural circadian rhythm of our bodies. We need food to stay healthy and to heal. Become aware of these rhythms and force yourself to wake up early and go to bed at a reasonable time, and to regulate your eating patterns. Doing so will keep the digestive system moving and provide you with the nutrients you need for both energy and healing.

PART 4: REDUCING/ELIMINATING AGGRAVANTS

*Synopsis: We will not heal if we keep completely derailing our efforts. Cut back as much as possible and search for healthy alternatives to your vices.*

Excessive coffee, espresso, cigarettes/tobacco, drugs, tea, wine, beer, liquor, milk (of any kind), sugary drinks, or over eating…all these things aggravate gastritis or bind up nutrients, impair digestion, or in some way wear on the body in ways counterproductive to healing. Chronic illness is not something that can be overcome half-heartedly. We may be doing everything right but still hold on to a vice or two, a secret "reward" that we indulge in every day. Such things are tolerable now and then, but small vices such as these on a daily basis can derail our journey back to health. Ironically, a lot of people with chronic health ailments turn to their vices more than they did when they were healthy.

The vice offers an outlet, a temporary escape from the doldrums of their illness.

Let's take coffee and espresso for example, which have been my particular weaknesses. Given the importance of hunger before eating, I often hold off on snacking or eating by simply drinking caffeinated beverages which I love, but over time I realized that these were holding me back in significant ways. Coffee and red wine are loaded with tannins, which are astringent, meaning they bind and curdle proteins, including the proteins on our tongue and on our stomach. Tannins act as "antinutrients," binding and inhibiting the absorption of nutrients, especially minerals, and aggravating the inflamed tissues within the digestive tract. Coffee, when combined with sugar and cream exacerbates gastritis in every possible way, increasing the porosity of the tissue and penetrability of acid into the blood.

I'll admit that unless you possess the most ardent, militaristic type of personality, it is extremely difficult to abandon all vices which may in some way block the road to recovering your health. The important thing is to cut back over time and limit how much you consume. Learn to take your coffee without sugar. Find varieties of your particular vice which might not be as aggravating. Darker, bolder coffee roasts actually have fewer tannins (as detected by the bitterness) than light roasts. Dry wines are less aggravating than sweeter varieties. Light beers with good carbonation are better than heavier, flatter beers. But over time strive to eliminate them altogether. These seemingly small shifts will ultimately mean the difference between healing completely and remaining chronically ill.

## PART 5: MAINTAIN A PHYSICALLY AND MENTALLY ACTIVE LIFESTYLE

*Synopsis: We were meant to be physically active and well oxygenated. Disease has a hard time taking hold when our bodies are oxygen-rich. The potential to live a meaningful, happy, and healthy life is a birthright, but it's up to us to achieve it. Engage the mind and body in some way every day; help yourself to help others.*

Our DNA contains the blueprints for us to lead active lives. Life was never meant to be spent sitting idly all day with no exercise. We're designed to be moving around outside, hunting and gathering our food, maintaining our shelters, building fires for heat, searching for resources and crafting tools that might better our lives. Being active outside everyday ensures that our blood is well oxygenated which empowers our immune systems and keeps our bodies alkaline – the fundamental precursor to strong health and healing. Being outside also ensures the exposure of our skin to sunlight, resulting in the production of vitamin D. Sunlight is also credited with improving everything from metabolism to blood pressure to cardiovascular health, immunity, digestion, and mood. An active lifestyle outdoors keeps our blood circulating, our bodies oxygenated, and our health strong.

Physical activity minimizes pockets of stagnation where disease can take hold. Stagnation and non-movement are the precursors to disease and death as much as poor diet and exposure to toxins. We are active by nature, and when we cultivate the discipline to become and remain active, our physical, emotional and spiritual well being align with the intentions of our design.

The key to developing an active lifestyle is consistency and baby steps. Ease into exercising every day and stay in your comfort zone until exercise becomes a part of your life, then worry about increasing the duration or intensity of that exercise. Even if you feel sick, are overweight, or are burdened with addictions of one sort or another, try to begin with 5 minutes a day of moderate exercise and stick to it. From that point you can build up and do more as you feel able, but never let a day go by without at least 5 minutes of moderate physical activity. Over time, 20 to 40 minutes of exercise a day will easily grow from that 5 minute minimum. A friend of mine used to remind me that if exercise could be in the form of a pill, it would be the most widely prescribed medication in the world.

It's also important to stay mentally stimulated as well. Mental stimulation isn't a luxury; it's a primary joy and the wonder of life. Our ancestors must have found daily stimulation through physical survival as hunter gatherers and through their social relationships and contemplation of the natural world. In this modern age, survival has become tied to earning an income, and the ways many people earn an income are completely devoid of mental stimulation. A life devoid of stimulation is an empty state of survival, a zombie-like existence driven only by the most basic desires.

Seek out meaningful relationships and pursue the interests that grab you and make them a priority in your life. If your employment grates on your soul, then search for a different kind of work even if it means making drastic changes. Above all I would say never restrict your experiences or ways of thinking by the expectations of others. Explore and develop your talents. By living mentally stimulating lives we have reasons to be healthy, which is the only way we can really help anyone else to become happy and healthy as well.

One final note to the reader on the process of recovering from illness: remember to always visualize recovering and living your life in a healthy state. It's been said that energy flows where attention goes, and it's far more effective to visualize the future you see yourself in than to constantly focus on your frustration and loathing of your discomfort. By focusing on illness and the negative aspects of one's life, those very aspects of life tend to manifest themselves day after day. Instead, lay the visual ground work for how your life will become, thereby providing your subconscious with a "map" to get there.

# 6

## *The Natural Diet...*

*Chapter synopsis: In its simplest terms, the natural diet for humans is what we would find locally in nature as omnivorous hunter-gatherers. Compared to today's western diet, there would be less grain and more fruits and vegetables.*

I don't want to put this forth as law because ultimately I do believe that everyone needs to discover for themselves what works and what doesn't through their own experimentation. In addition, what one person can eat that may be completely natural, another person may have trouble with, especially in cases of common allergens such as gluten or shellfish or peanuts.

What follows are the foods I believe comprise the natural human diet. Beginning at birth, the natural human diet starts with the mother's raw, fresh breast milk – a non-replicable powerhouse of nutrients and immune system cofactors that help prime the child's immune system and establish proper beneficial bacteria in the colon. At least for the first few weeks or months, breast milk is very important and is something I don't believe any "formula" can fully take the place of. From that point on, essentially the natural diet includes any whole food, naturally raised or grown in organic soils, and preferably local.

## I. Wild or Free Range Organic Meat, Fish and Poultry

As discussed in the nutrition crash course, our health depends on the inclusion of eight essential amino acids in our diet. These are the building blocks of the non-essential amino acids and every protein in our body. The plant kingdom is weak in supplying these essential amino acids, especially lyseine and methionine. Furthermore, people with compromised digestion and an imbalance of beneficial colonic bacteria will have even greater trouble extracting the amino acids from the tough fibers of their plant sources such as beans and whole grains.

Wild or free range/organic fish and meats are more balanced in fatty acids that temper or reduce inflammation (including Omega-3 fatty acids) as opposed to the inflammatory effects of meats from animals raised in toxic environments. When the ultra distance runner Dean Karnazes (who once ran 350 miles without stopping) was asked, "If there were one healthy food item that you had to eat every day, what would it be?" his answer was "Wild Pacific salmon."

Finally, animal meat and fish, when cooked properly and eaten when hungry, has the unique ability to trigger the primordial pathway of Active Digestion – a factor in maximizing digestive power and healing from chronic illness.

## II. Fruits and Vegetables (raw and cooked)

Fruits and vegetables play the greatest role in alkalizing your body and are crucial to rebuilding your healing power. The minerals you get from fruits and vegetables are the building blocks of everything else in your body, and make no mistake, it is minerals that will ultimately empower you with strong digestion (which you will *feel*), and a strong and alkaline body. Minerals are the "salt of the earth," and they come directly from the soil in which vegetables and fruits grow. There is simply no substitute for an abundance of vegetables (and fruits, though they are calorie rich and less alkalizing than most vegetables) in terms of obtaining the minerals we need for health and healing.

Prior to modern concepts of nutrition, fruits and vegetables were all just "plants" to our hunter-gatherer ancestors. In fact, the primary difference between most fruits and vegetables is only sugar content and texture. Fruits are generally softer and sweeter depending on their ripeness, while vegetables are less sweet and hardier. Otherwise, per weight, most fruits and vegetables are equally nutritious in vitamin, mineral, and fiber content. Raw fruits and vegetables (i.e., not heated above 118 degrees F at which point proteins and enzymes begin to denature), grown organically or in the wild, introduce beneficial bacteria as well as a level of vitamins and phytonutrients that would otherwise perish in cooking. However, lightly cooked vegetables and some fruits are easier for the body to digest and are easier to assimilate minerals and other nutrients from. Therefore, a combination of cooked and raw fruits and vegetables comprise the optimum and natural diet for the human body.

## III. Organic Eggs and dairy

As omnivorous hunter-gatherers, eggs would have been a natural and nutritionally rich part of our ancestral diet. In addition, milk found in the digestive systems of young hunted mammals would have been a gem of nutrients, although fresh liquid milk did not come about until the agricultural revolution only 10,000 years ago. While fresh liquid milk is often difficult for people to digest because of the protein and/or lactose it contains, curdled and partially digested/fermented milk in the guts of young mammals would have been much easier for humans to digest, raw or cooked. Raw curdled milk also is a rich source of live, active probiotic bacteria.

Cheese can be really helpful in triggering AD when cooked/melted but it can also trigger PD if raw or soft. Composed primarily of fat and protein, cheese qualifies as APF but when eaten raw it tends to mix with saliva, coat and buffer the stomach wall from acid, and trigger PD. When cooked, however, the proteins in cheese denature (proteins are like bundled strings that can unravel or fold up in the presence of heat or acid) and contract while the fat melts and is squeezed out of the protein matrix, hence the oiliness of melted cheese. Fatty acids in the oils are detected in the duodenum and trigger AD. Firmer cheeses are better than softer ones since they tend to release their oils more when melted. Melted cheese doesn't mix with saliva the way raw cheese does, but remains more of a solid mass and sinks in the stomach, allowing the oils to be detected in the duodenum, triggering AD. Therefore as a general rule, melted cheese is good (when hungry for it, of course) while raw cheese is either neutral or troublesome in excess but can be included in small amounts with other foods as a rich probiotic source. Processed cheeses (which hardly release oils when melted) are never good and don't trigger AD.

**IV. Whole Grains, Seeds, and Starches**

Whole grains are nutritional powerhouses, loaded with vitamins and minerals and slow-release carbohydrates that keep us satisfied and keep cravings at bay. Grains are simply the seeds of grasses, and hunter-gatherers would have found these sources of energy throughout the world. However, some grains contain a protein called *gluten* that can trigger allergic reactions in people with celiac disease. These grains include wheat, oats, barley, and rye.

Other seeds such as legumes are harder to digest, but provide large amounts of fiber and are nutritionally rich in amino acids and minerals. However, legumes also contain powerful anti-nutrients that are deactivated during sprouting and/or cooking, and their high plant protein content can trigger allergic reactions in people as well. For example peanuts, which are a type of legume, contain a common allergen which can cause extreme reactions and even death in some people. Fatty seeds such as pumpkin and sunflower seeds and nuts are rich in magnesium and other trace minerals but very difficult to digest, so are best eaten sparingly, sprinkled on other foods or mixed in with salads or grains.

Starch sources such as tubers (potatoes, sweet potatoes, yams, etc) and starchy fruits (bananas, plantains, breadfruit) are extremely rich in potassium and vitamin C, and low in potentially allergenic proteins that grains and seeds tend to have. These non-seed sources of carbohydrates have been dietary staples for indigenous peoples throughout the world for millennia, and remain so today.

All whole food starches also provide a food source for the beneficial bacteria in our guts which are indispensable in healing and maintaining our overall health.

## V. Leafy greens and seaweed

Virtually all land animals, including carnivores, ingest leafy greens from time to time and humans are no exception. Leafy greens such as spinach, kale, romaine lettuce and arugula impart powerful health benefits that strengthen our digestion and radically reduce inflammation throughout the body. This is especially true for gastritis, and the reason I consider raw leafy greens to be "nature's medicine." Greens cool our bodies and stimulate AD which helps with stomach emptying and breaking up of digestive stagnation.

Seaweed is one of the most mineral-rich and alkalizing foods on the planet. Adding seaweed such as kelp or dulse to soups and salads will ensure your body gets a solid boost of both macro minerals and trace minerals, as well as a host of nutrients that will boost immunity and overall health.

## VI. Spices, ferments, and acids

Cayenne pepper and other hot peppers: One of the most unique and helpful spices available. Cayenne adds heat and stimulates mucus secretion in the stomach which protects the inflamed tissue. It can be counterproductive when used in excess, but when added to most foods it irritates the stomach lining just enough to stimulate self-protective measures which in turn are beneficial to healing from gastritis. Furthermore, cayenne and other hot peppers contain antiviral, antibiotic and antifungal compounds and are one of the richest food sources of vitamin C available. Of course such small amounts are eaten that their vitamin and mineral content should not be considered too relevant.

All other plant spices (ginger, turmeric, pepper, herbs, etc) and alcoholic ferments used as spices in food prep can stimulate digestion and impart anti-inflammatory and anti-viral properties. They also help break up stagnation and offer trace minerals and nutrients that greatly aid in healing. Don't get carried away with any one particular spice (other than perhaps cayenne) but learn to use a variety of them frequently in food preparation and collectively they will play an important role in maximizing health and healing.

Alcohols and ferments made from whole food sources such as wine from grapes or mead from fruits and honey, or beer from whole grains are a completely natural part of the diet in moderation. Alcohols such as wine or beer can add digestion-stimulating properties to meals and, in moderation, alcohol thins the blood and helps dissolve cholesterol in the arteries. All ferments including soya sauce, yogurt, raw vinegar, and alcohol add digestion stimulating flavor as well, but it's best to limit them to a small but consistent part of the diet. Raw fermented foods in general are teaming with probiotics and are essential for full health and recovering from illness. Probiotics in their natural food substrates can survive digestion and gradually build up and maintain healthy colonies in the lower digestive system. However, if these colonies aren't well fed (I know, it sounds strange) with plenty of fruit, vegetable, and whole grain fiber, then they will not be able to establish and maintain themselves.

Acids such as lemon juice, lime juice, vinegar, etc, can help lower the pH of food and ward off a stomach acid rebound reaction and PD. Add lemon juice to other juices, vegetables, fruits, soups, and other foods to enhance their flavor, increase their acidity and ward off PD.

In summary, humans have always been omnivorous hunter-gatherers, and ever since we learned to make and control fire, we've used it to cook some of our food, especially hardy plant foods and most animal foods. In preparing the whole foods from our natural diet, remember to employ the "keys to food preparation" outlined in chapter four, which in summary are:

- Keep meats and APF foods separate enough from other foods, sauces, dressings and condiments so they're recognizable to the digestive system as APF.
- Use sauces, condiments and dressings in minimal amounts. Learn to flavor with acids and spices more than sugars.

- Don't overcook grains or starches.

Also keep in mind that the foods listed here in the Natural Diet are the ideal "gold standard" of what we would naturally be putting into our bodies. This doesn't mean that including some slightly processed or nonlocal foods here and there will completely undermine the benefits of moving in the direction of this diet. The trick is to move subtly but consistently in the direction of a more healthy and natural diet over time. In a nutshell, this simply means switching over to organic and free range meats and animal foods while increasing the amount of fruits and vegetables and reducing the amount of processed foods in the diet.

Maintaining a 100% organic, natural, pure diet can be extremely expensive unless you live on a farm or in the wilderness. If you're like me and don't have much money, it pays to prioritize what foods are worth the extra buck. In general, I put animal products such as meat, fish, eggs, and dairy at the top of the list to spend a little extra for. Not only are naturally raised animal foods free of toxins and unhealthy fats (and full of healthy ones), but it's also nice knowing that I'm not contributing to the suffering of animals raised in inhumane conditions.

Beyond animal products, whole food starches such as grains, potatoes, tubers or bananas are all quite affordable and far more nutritious and alkalizing than processed flour products. Fruits and vegetables that aren't organic are still loaded with minerals and nutrients and are better than no fruits or vegetables at all. The trick to increasing your fruit and vegetable intake while maintaining your budget is to minimize waste. Since produce perishes relatively quickly (unless frozen), by planning meals ahead and buying only what you need, you can better ensure that your grocery money doesn't end up in the garbage. An obvious concept, but one that still requires practice and discipline to master!

## 7

## *Meal Ideas to Get Started...*

*"Let thy food be thy medicine, and thy medicine be thy food" –
Hippocrates*

I'm not much of a cook, so what follows are some basic suggestions to get you started. There are many excellent cookbooks that offer simple, easy to prepare, and delicious meal ideas focused on everything from methods of cooking (grilling, roasting, slow cooking) to specific ingredients (poultry, beef, vegetarian, vegan) to cultural dishes (Indian, Japanese, Mediterranean, Italian) to meals that can be prepared in 15 minutes or less. The only thing you have to do is pick out the recipes that conform to what you now know to be healing and empowering. Also check in at www.overcomeillness.net for meal recipe updates in the near future.

The beauty of healing through understanding the concepts of Active Digestion and Passive Digestion is that the ingredients and meals you can prepare are virtually limitless, so long as you follow the basic rules of food preparation and follow your hunger. The hard part, at least for anyone who doesn't particularly enjoy cooking (like me), is actually doing it. This is why it's important to start with simple meals and ways of preparing meats and vegetables that are tasty and not too time-consuming.

Once again, here's what you have to watch out for:

1. Eating when not hungry
2. Excessive oil, sauces, dressings, or marinades (especially if sweet or thick)
3. Overly pasty (overcooked potatoes or grains) or fluffy, flour based starches (cake, pancakes, etc.).
4. Thick soups (brothy soups are OK)

Here's what you should strive for:

1. Eat when hungry – strong hunger alone is an AD stimulant
2. Balanced, filling meals with cooked, non-matrix APF (that is, not "hidden" in thick sauces or excessive starch) such as melted butter, melted cheese, roasted fish or meats, along with vegetables both raw and lightly cooked, and wholesome starches, etc. Use just enough sauce or dressings to flavor, never excess.
3. Include a side salad of fresh leafy greens at least once a day.
4. Flavor with spices including cayenne often, and increase acidity of foods to taste with lemon, lime, or vinegar to stave off rebound acid secretion and PD.

Some of the things I like for breakfast if I'm hungry are:

- Leftovers! Soups (with hot sauce or lemon to taste) with a toasted bagel are good, but any balanced meal that was lunch or dinner a day or two before makes a great breakfast as well.
- Organic bacon or sausage, eggs (over medium), potatoes fried in leftover grease (flavored with salt and vinegar/hot sauce) or bagel toasted with butter. You can add a small amount of cooked spinach as well to further alkalize the body if desired, with a little lemon or vinegar.
- Crepes (whole white flour mixed with milk to runny consistency, ladled onto a hot pan quite thin and cooked well through). Add butter and honey, small amounts of fruit or some raw yogurt and lemon juice, or whatever else sounds good. A little melted cheese can be good too.
- Whole grain pancakes can be tolerable only when very hungry and with plenty of fresh, tart fruit cooked in. I like to mix in a bunch of fresh blueberries in the batter before cooking.
- Mixed chopped fruits. Add citrus, pineapple, or lemon to increase acidity.
- Oatmeal is great, but be sure not to overcook. Steel cut, traditional, or quick 1-minute are all whole grain oats but just have different cooking times. Flavor with berries (which add a

little acidic tartness along with an abundance of minerals and vitamins) and just enough honey to taste. Tolerable without APF when hungry.

- An omelet with any combination of vegetables, cheese and/or meat.
- If craving a sugar boost, drink orange juice or other acidic or tart fruit juice but watered down to around 50/50 or to "just sweet enough."
- A bowl of cereal is tolerable once in a while but liquid milk is very buffering and triggers rebound acid and PD, so use just enough milk to coat and ideally add a little acidic juicy fruits such as blueberries or strawberries to drop the pH a bit. All the more important that the next meal is balanced with APF and/or raw greens.

If NOT very hungry, just stick with diluted juice or juicy fruit until you build up hunger for something more substantial.

Some things that work for lunch or dinner include:

- Buffalo (as in spicy "buffalo" sauce – not buffalo the animal) chicken sandwich (minimal bread to avoid APF "matrix"), French fries (with salt, vinegar, or buffalo sauce...try to avoid ketchup in all things), side salad.

- Spicy beef chili (with a little bread if desired). This is a nutrition grenade packed with vitamins, minerals, protein, fiber (from beans), but it is dense. Make a lot and keep it on hand or frozen.
- Simple roast beef, turkey, or ham sandwich with sharp cheddar cheese, pickles or hot peppers (add acidity), baby greens, and minimal condiments to taste. Whole white or Italian bread is easier to digest than whole wheat and is less of a PD trigger.
- Meatballs made with 85-90% lean ground free range, organic meat of any kind are excellent to have on hand and are really easy to make. There are hundreds of meatball recipes, but use only wholesome ingredients if possible bake them covered so they don't dry out.
- Spaghetti (whole grain) with sauce "cooked in" and meatballs made with organic meat, egg, and seasoning and a side salad. (Fast food and store-bought meatballs are often mostly textured vegetable protein filler and a million other ingredients that aren't natural and healthy APF)
- Pizza topped with other healthy vegetables/meats works really well, especially with hot peppers and a side salad.
- Burgers with organic, free range meat. The fat in such meat is perfectly good for you. If you can't find quality burger meat, most stores will grind any cut of meat into burger meat for you. Go easy on the condiments, and balance with a side salad.

- Homemade fries – chop up a potato and bake with olive oil and sea salt and other herbs or spices to taste.
- Salmon with a little mayonnaise and mustard on top, baked at 350 for 20 minutes, is super easy, tasty, and anti-inflammatory. Add rice or roasted potatoes (with oil, lemon and oregano) and roasted or lightly steamed vegetables with salt and lemon.
- Side salad with dark leafy greens and a little feta cheese (raw feta is a good source of probiotics). If anything can be considered "medicine" in the NDL, it is raw leafy greens! Spinach, romaine lettuce, or baby greens all work well. Mix in with a little iceberg lettuce for crunch if you want.

Including small amounts of unpasteurized, raw cheeses in salads or in sandwiches is a good way to get live, active probiotics into the diet, along with all the other nutrients of the cheese itself.

Desserts:

Desserts are risky unless you eat them on a hungry, empty stomach or after a balanced AD-triggering meal. Desserts that are mostly fruit based with fresh and acidic or tart fruits such as strawberry-rhubarb pie and thinner crust and less "gunky" fillings are ideal in minimizing PD and rebound acid.  Beware of store-bought pies which the food industry loads with cheap filler and minimal, low quality fruits.

Puddings and creamy deserts tend to trigger PD, but are tolerable in small amounts after an AD meal.  Remember also that cravings for potentially risky desserts can be minimized simply by filling up on a balanced, AD-triggering meal.

Drinks and Snacks:

Just remember, the sweeter the drink the more acidic it should be, so add lemon or dilute with water.  Sweet drinks should be made from tart or acidic fruit juices such as cranberry juice, orange juice, or grapefruit juice.

While coffee is not part of the NDL, if you must have your coffee, opt for darker, less bitter roasts and work on eliminating your taste for sugar.  Better yet, opt for tea with a little honey as a natural sweetener.  Every once in, at the extreme end of the spectrum, a natural soda such as Ginger Ale is tolerable but eating balanced meals will minimize cravings for super sweet drinks like soda.

Fruits and fruit-starch-fat combinations such as leftover desserts make great snacks but don't rule out raw vegetables like carrots or broccoli and a dip such as spicy tomato or black bean salsa or hummus (add lemon!).  Salsa and whole grain, low fat corn chips or other whole grain chips are a good choice too.

I hope that at least gets you started. Get your hands on a few good recipe books or magazines, or do your best to teach the cook in your house how to prepare food that will help you and not hurt you. It's also always a good idea to make enough for leftovers that you can eat the next day, or that you can freeze and have ready for when you're hungry but have nothing prepared.

Fast food and dining out choices:

If you're in a situation where you need to eat at a fast food restaurant or dine out, what you've learned in this guide should enable you to be ok. Remember that the meats and ingredients at nearly all restaurant chains (fast food or not) are the lowest possible quality. Burgers are soaked in grease, so take a couple napkins and squeeze some of that grease out. If a burger or sandwich comes in a huge bun or too much bread, remember bread hinders detection of APF and AD, so get rid of excessive bread (sometimes I eat burgers with only one side of the bun) or balance with an AD stimulating salad.

For more meal ideas I will try and get a recipe section going on my website (the address is listed on the inside of the first page) in the near future...

# 8

## *Healing on Restricted Diets*

*It's harder, but not impossible*

The following are examples of restricted diets that people may be on for one reason or another. Obviously I don't encourage these diets but I also realize people are different. Whether you believe strongly in the ideals of a diet or are limited by allergies or are living amongst others who maintain a restricted diet (for example, with a host family abroad), then here are some ways to maximize the healing powers of such diets.

VEGETARIAN DIET

If you're a lacto-ovo vegetarian, meaning you don't eat meat but you're not opposed to eggs or dairy, remember that melted cheese and melted butter are still APF and help trigger AD. Use these to your advantage when hungry for them. As a vegetarian, you will need to make a special effort to avoid the aggravating foods, drinks and excessively thick sauces and soups. Emphasize alkalizing vegetables (lightly steamed or raw), raw leafy greens, and live active probiotic cultures to build up your lower digestive strength.

VEGAN DIET

Vegans will have a tough time since they eat no animal source foods whatsoever. Raw leafy greens and hunger are your best allies in triggering AD. Spices are essential, especially cayenne pepper, which will maintain your protective mucus lining. Spices and ferments (cooking with some white wine, for example) also tend to stimulate digestion so make foods as flavorful and delicious as possible!

RAW FOOD DIET

Raw foods are foods that have not been heated past 118 degrees Fahrenheit, the temperature at which proteins begin to denature. Proteins are the building blocks of enzymes, which raw food dieters believe are one of the keys to good health. If you are a raw food purist, you have your work cut out for you not just in maintaining the diet but in healing from chronic illness. If you're a raw food omnivore and APF is still an option so long as it's raw, then I would sterilize (with acid such as lemon juice, or vinegar, or spices) meat and dehydrate it similar to beef jerky (which is sometimes also smoked). Raw butter is fair game, and I believe even melts at a temperature less than 118 degrees. Raw leafy greens are on your side, as are plenty of alkalizing vegetables and fruits and soaked whole grains, etc. Since many raw foods tend to have a high water content, dehydration helps meals and snacks become more filling and in some cases more easily digestible. Also raw vegetables can be harder to digest than lightly cooked vegetables so it's important to chew everything extremely well on a raw food diet. Make use of that upper temperature; 118 degrees is actually quite warm, and soaking grains around that temperature will expedite the process of gelatinizing the starches and can even be served warm as well. You can even have tea and warm drinks on a raw diet.

INGREDIENT RESTRICTED DIETS

If you have celiac disease and can't eat gluten, or other allergies that restrict certain foods from your diet, just follow the natural diet to the best of your ability while steering clear of your allergic triggers. Use the diet and food preparation guidelines to develop a delicious and diverse menu with the ingredients you can use, and you should be fine.

# 9

## *The End Game*

*From managing to curing chronic illness*

The causes of chronic illness can run deep and recovery can take some time. Depending on the severity of your disease and your ability to adhere to the natural diet and lifestyle, you can expect a return to normal levels of energy and well being sometime between a few days to a few months. But the management of chronic illness is always subject to relapse, and relapse tends to happen more often without the help and support of others.

Once you understand how to prepare meals that will empower the innate healing potential of your body, the next step is to actually DO it. In a way, you must become a modern day hunter-gatherer. For so many reasons maintaining a healing diet is easier said than done. It requires a continuing, concerted focus to successfully pull off. Allot a certain amount of time every day for gathering the ingredients you will need and 'hunting' down quality, organic meats or fish that you can use to prepare your next few meals. I've learned that it's mentally easier when you think of a task in terms of time. "Preparing dinner" can sound overwhelming to anyone unaccustomed to cooking, but when you say to yourself, "in 15 minutes I'll be done," or "in 30 minutes I'll be done," suddenly doing the task becomes easier.

The good news is the more you work at it, the easier and more habitual the path to healing will become. As your energy and health improve over time, you will find it easier to let go of the habits that impair your health and replace them with healthier, life-affirming foods, drinks, and activities.

It's up to you to make those around you or those you live with aware of your needs. Not doing so is not only unhelpful to you, it's unhelpful to them. Those to whom you are close will indirectly benefit from your well-being or to an extent, suffer with you. In turn, by observing or participating in your shift to a natural diet, their health will directly benefit as well. The natural diet is not a limiting one; it's a diet that is specific to subtle details in food preparation and natural, quality ingredients and therefore can be enjoyed by all.

Over time, as one gets stronger and the body adjusts to deeper levels of health and balance, there will eventually be a point when you can live as you lived before developing the illness; you'll be cured. It won't be the immediate and dramatic symptom suppression type "cure" we've come to expect from prescription drugs and the medical industry but will be our body curing the illness in its own good time. But the human body is not indestructible, and being cured does not mean that you can't get sick again. Therefore, maintaining a healthy diet and lifestyle should not be a temporary endeavor but a lifelong goal.

## 10

# *Health Misunderstanding and Myths*

*Don't always believe what you always hear*

Over the years I've found there to be an abundance of health myths that are alive and well in society at large, from needing eight glasses of water a day to the inflated importance of milk in the diet to the importance of milk NOT in the diet, to the unhealthiness of red meat and fat in general to the notion that dietary cholesterol is responsible for the level of cholesterol in our bodies, and so forth and so on. All these ideas leave people confused and sick. My goal here is to tackle just a few of them (in no particular order) in hopes that I will save people a few agonizing weeks or months of adhering to ideas that were never helpful because they were never fully true to begin with. I say "fully" true because there is some validity to almost every health claim out there, including contradictory ones where, for example, a certain food is good for you but an excess of that food is also not good for you. The following "myths" I refer to in the more extreme degrees to which they're advocated as true.

## "Food Combining"

There have been many books written and advice dispensed by health professionals on how to combine and not combine ingredients in meals for optimal digestion. The basic reasoning goes like this: carbohydrates (starches and sugars) require alkaline digestive fluids which are produced in the mouth and in the duodenum/small intestine and are digested quickly. Protein requires acid to break down and digests slowly. Fats digest slowly. Therefore, it's important to not combine quick digesting foods that require alkaline digestive fluids with slowly digesting foods that require acid, or they will neutralize each other and not digest well and ferment in your gut. Vegetables are said to be "neutral" and can be combined with either starches or proteins.

I attempted to follow these food combining "rules" for a long time and found them to be quite unsustainable. This is NOT to say that you should mix and match anything out there in the strangest combinations imaginable and not worry about it. Indeed, simple food combinations do seem to digest better than extremely complex ones. However, the stalling the breakdown of starch by the acidity of the stomach is only temporary. As food moves into the duodenum, starches, fats, and proteins are fully broken down during Active Digestion. Recall that in Active Digestion, proteins, fats, and carbohydrates are all mixed with powerful digestive enzymes and have the rest of the digestive tract to be broken down and absorbed. So combining meats and starches is not much of an issue. Combining small amounts of fruit and juices with other foods to flavor or taste also isn't a problem, so long as you follow your hunger signals and don't overdo it.

The important thing with regard to food combining comes back to simply eating balanced meals when hungry, and not stuffing yourself to excess. As hunter gatherers, we snacked as we foraged and hunted, but we also ate socially at times, and what was hunted and gathered was shared.

### "The Herxheimer Reaction"

The *Herxheimer Reaction* refers to the horrible feeling of grogginess and fatigue that follows soon after commencing a fast or a cleanse. The idea is that when we stop eating, our bodies have a chance to finally "clean house" at the cellular level and dislodge all kinds of toxins that have accumulated over time. Another idea is that the bacteria or yeast that had been infecting us die off and release toxins which make us feel lousy. In some cases, the Herxheimer reaction can be so intense that it can cause organ failure and even death in people who are overweight or extremely sick.

While I believe there's some truth to the idea of the Herxheimer reaction occurring in people who are obese or have maintained very unhealthy, toxic lifestyles, there's another reason for feeling lousy when we stop eating. What actually happens when we stop eating food is that our digestive system shuts down, and toxins and acid in the body that normally exit through the digestive system stall and stagnate within the body. These aren't necessarily toxins that have been stagnating in the body all along, they are toxins that are being released by the cells from normal cellular metabolism, and they have nowhere to go!

In my experience, the best and "cleanest" I feel is when I eat wholesome, balanced meals on a regular basis. Not only do these meals provide the energy and nutrients the body needs on a daily basis, but they cleanse the body by providing fiber and bulk which binds toxins and carries them out of the body. The fat in meals stimulates gallbladder contraction which squeezes out all the bile in the gallbladder, warding off the possible formation of gallstones from stagnating bile.

From an evolutionary standpoint, our bodies are the cleanest and most efficient when we eat wholesome balanced meals on a regular basis and stay physically active and get plenty of fresh air. "Cleaning house" isn't something our bodies do now and then. It's something our bodies do constantly and efficiently, so long as we're eating and living naturally. This comes up again in the myth of *The Cleanse* later on.

### *The Cholesterol Myth*

It's widely assumed that if you have high cholesterol, you should lay off dietary cholesterol such as butter and juicy burgers and bacon.

This isn't true. What's needed instead is an increase in fiber (both soluble and insoluble) along with meals that include cholesterol and fats in order to bind cholesterol and bile acids and carry them out of the system.

The body NEEDS cholesterol for thousands of reasons...and if it doesn't get it through diet, our liver will compensate and increase production. It's possible that if we don't get enough cholesterol in the diet, our liver will overcompensate in production. When this happens, cholesterol levels can get out of control.

Without question, exercise is a primary factor in reducing arterial cholesterol. The powerful pumping of blood during exercise literally wears away and dislodges cholesterol in the arteries. So increased fiber and exercise are the primary factors in reducing one's cholesterol, NOT decreasing or eliminating dietary cholesterol intake (although as with everything, it shouldn't be consumed excessively either).

*Gallbladder Disease*

Gallbladder removal surgery (cholecystectomy) is a common practice today, with over 500,000 operations annually in the United States. The reason for these operations is the presence of gallstones or a diseased and infected gallbladder.

The gallbladder is a small sack directly under the liver that stores bile and secretes it to break down fat in the duodenum (as in Active Digestion). In the natural diet and lifestyle of our ancestors, fatty and rich foods were encountered sporadically and when they were, our bodies needed the digestive power to efficiently process those foods. The gallbladder stores bile for just such occasions, and when fat was eaten, it was usually eaten in large amounts, stimulating the gallbladder to contract violently and squeeze out all the stored bile.

However, if the gallbladder is rarely stimulated to contract, as would happen in people who have adopted low fat diets, or is constantly stimulated (by a constant intake of fatty foods) and therefore never contracts with its full potential, then bile stagnates in the gallbladder. Over time, this leads to the formation and enlargement of gallstones. Eventually, a stone can enter the common bile duct during bile secretion, causing a painful gallbladder attack.

Gallbladder surgery in extreme cases is necessary. But without the gallbladder, the liver constantly leaks bile into the small intestine, leading to things such as decreased metabolism and diarrhea. Meanwhile, the underlying problem of sluggish bile flow remains. If bile flow is sluggish, stones can even form in the liver.

Before rushing to have your gallbladder removed, try to determine just how bad the stones are by consulting with your doctor, and look into alternative ways to deal with minor gallstones (such as the gallbladder flush) while making appropriate changes to achieve a more natural diet and lifestyle. By shifting to more balanced meals with APF and limiting snacking, the gallbladder will begin to function as it was meant to.

### The *"Weak LES" in Gastroesophogal Reflux Disease (GERD)*

If you or someone you know has ever experienced a bout of acid reflux, you know it's not pleasant. Acid from the stomach splashes into the esophagus and burns. Indigestion and inability to sleep are commonly associated with acid reflux, which for some people can be chronic.

The experts' explanation: a "weak" lower esophageal sphincter (LES) muscle, the muscle that closes the lower esophagus and separates it from the stomach. But that's like saying the cause of the United States dropping the atomic bomb on Hiroshima was the opening of the bay doors on the B-29 the weapon. In both cases there are other, deeper reasons involved. Yes, the lower esophageal sphincter is open when it shouldn't be, but why is it open?

I believe the real cause of acid reflux is not too much acid and a weak LES but too little acid. Closing of the LES depends on strong acid signaling it to close and protect the lower esophagus. While acid reflux is painful, the acid is still not as concentrated as it needs to be to signal the LES to remain tightly closed. Therefore, the way to heal GERD is to cut back on excessive sweets that compete with acid for binding sites on pH detector proteins ("tricking" the stomach into ignoring the actual acid concentration, as described earlier in chapter four) as well as cutting back on acid buffers such as milk and creamy sauces and dressings. Here again a more natural diet will do wonders. Eat regular spaced, balanced meals, letting hunger be your guide, and include APF and greens to stimulate Active Digestion and shift the digestive burden down to the duodenum.

*"Bananas for Potassium, Milk for Calcium,
& Orange Juice for Vitamin C"*

Bananas are rich in potassium but hardly more than nearly every other fruit and vegetable out there and are actually lower than many per calorie. For example, a medium tomato has as much potassium as a banana but only a fraction of the calories. When reduced to tomato sauce or tomato paste, tomatoes both far outperform bananas in potassium density. Cantaloupe is loaded with potassium. But compared to other fruits, bananas are uniquely high in vitamin B and magnesium, two nutrients that have a particularly calming effect.

Milk is high in calcium, but so are cruciferous vegetables such as kale and broccoli, whole sesame seeds, sardines (with bones), and many other natural whole foods. More important, the calcium in these foods is easier to absorb than the calcium in milk.

Vitamin C is abundant in virtually all fruits and vegetables. Orange juice is rich in it but is also very high in sugars, making orange juice somewhat poor in vitamin C on a per-calorie basis. Leafy greens, broccoli, and many other vegetables out-perform orange juice in the vitamin C-per-calorie department.

### "Calcium for Osteoperosis"

Osteoporosis is a weakening of the bones due to mineral loss. Calcium is a major mineral in bones, along with phosphorous. However, the problem isn't a lack of calcium in the diet per se. The problem is that the modern western diet lacks micronutrients in general and is excessively high in processed foods that cause the body to be excessively acidic. To neutralize this acid, the body leaches calcium and alkaline minerals from the bones.

The milk industry wants you to drink more milk, and has pulled every string possible to make the public think that osteoporosis is a direct result of not drinking enough milk and getting enough calcium. However, evidence to the contrary exists in societies all around the globe who have more wholesome diets in which milk is hardly consumed at all. These societies have far lower rates of osteoporosis than those of us in the West. Their diets, mineral rich and balanced with whole foods have the effect of alkalizing the body and strengthening the bones.

## "The Cleanse"

Cleanses seem to be all the rage these days. In my experience with cleanses, the idea that people have all kinds of toxic sludge caked to the walls of their digestive systems and in their cells and blood that can only be eliminated by a strict diet of some sort, perhaps only fruits or vegetables or juice or water, is a bit extreme. But more important, cleanses are not sustainable and often only lead to a rebound indulgence in the exact foods that were avoided in the cleanse itself. At worst, extreme cleanses can deprive us of important nutrients and compromise the balance of our digestive flora (especially when it comes to "colonic cleanses").

Our DNA holds the blueprints for our bodies to exist in a healthy and clean state throughout our lives. I believe the cleanest we can be is by simply eating when we're hungry and consuming wholesome and healthy foods with plenty of fiber and bulk. By eating a variety of foods with the full range of nutrients including APF, cravings are avoided, and toxins and waste are bound in the bulky fiber of whole plant foods and flushed from the system. This provides abundant energy for daily exercise, which increases circulation and breaks up stagnation. We cannot be cleaner than when we're eating naturally and only when we're hungry and exercising on a daily basis.

**11**

# *Recovering from other Chronic Illnesses through the Natural Diet and Lifestyle...*

*Chapter synopsis: In my view all chronic diseases can be traced to a deviation from our natural way of living, with the end result being an increase in acid/toxins and a decrease in nutrients and circulation. By changing how we live back to a natural state (described in chapter five) we can avoid and reverse chronic disease.*

As I mentioned earlier in this guide, I believe the fundamental trigger of disease is excess acid/toxins in the blood and/or insufficient nutrients/oxygen. The origins of these imbalances are poor diet and/or insufficient exercise or rest, which leads to weakness, infection, and the cascade of chronic illness. I believe recovering from these illnesses will require a return to the NDL.

For every disease I discuss in this chapter, there is obviously an entire field dedicated to its study and the development of treatments. What follows is only my own in-depth look at a few illnesses from the standpoint that, despite billions of dollars of research, science has yet to produce a cure or to even prove the pathways by which the diseases manifest themselves. I offer my own beliefs on the causes of some of the major illnesses plaguing society today, and how living in accordance with the NDL can mitigate and reverse those causes. Society in general and the healthcare industry in particular have become deeply invested in common, accepted understandings of many illnesses, whether those views stand on a solid foundation of proof or not.

When I decided out of curiosity to research how HIV causes AIDS, I had trouble finding any clear explanation of how the virus caused the disease. As I looked deeper, I found myself reading about what appeared to be scientifically valid skepticism of the entire HIV-AIDS paradigm. Aware of my own lack of expertise on the subject and convinced there was something that I was missing, I emailed professors of virology and biochemistry at a prominent university and asked them to enlighten me on why the AIDS "dissidents" were wrong. To my great surprise, they offered no clear repudiation of the questions regarding the connection between HIV and AIDS, and when I respectfully pressed them a little more, I was essentially told that we would have to "agree to disagree." This was shocking. How could an issue as massive as HIV-AIDS boil down to opinion? To this day I remain fascinated by the possibility that HIV-AIDS might be an enormous misunderstanding, and hopeful that sufferers of the diseases classified under AIDS might regain their health through lifestyle and dietary modifications.

I also realize the importance to one's credibility of not getting lumped in with conspiracy theorists who question ideas without sufficient expertise to do so. However, history is well peppered with instances where the beliefs of a vast majority were exposed as false, and ultimately I think it's the responsibility of every individual to take a look at the evidence and decide for themselves what may or may not be true.

## HIV-AIDS

AIDS, or Acquired Immunodeficiency Syndrome, is an extremely political illness with a historically fluid definition. Recall that a "syndrome" is a collection of symptoms that are grouped together under the umbrella of a single name or diagnosis. When AIDS was first named back in the early 1980's, it referred primarily to individuals with very low immunity who were infected with Pneumocystis Carinii Pneumonia (PCP, a lung infection) or Kaposi's Sarcoma (a rare skin cancer).

Within a few years, the US Centers for Disease Control (CDC) had expanded the definition of AIDS to include over a dozen "indicator diseases" combined with diminished immunity. Then, in 1987, the CDC broadened the definition to increase the number of indicator diseases of AIDS by about a third, and again in 1992 to bring the total number of AIDS indicator diseases to 29.

**The definition of AIDS today is the presence of any one of 29 indicator diseases with a positive HIV antibody test result**. If a person is HIV negative, they do not have AIDS but just the indicator disease. As the conditions for an AIDS diagnosis changed, it allowed a wider and wider net to be cast over the number of people suffering from the syndrome, supporting the fear and conviction of its viral etiology.

Unlike other discoveries of viruses that have been determined to cause certain diseases, there has never been a scientific paper or group of papers published that proves the link between HIV and AIDS. Instead, the notion that HIV was the cause of AIDS was announced, literally, at a press conference in Washington, D.C. on April 23, 1984. Margaret Heckly, then the secretary of Health and Human Services, announced that a scientist named Robert Gallo and his colleagues had discovered a virus that was the "probable" cause of AIDS. And with that, the cat was out of the bag.

The ability of people to be convinced of and believe in a myth, support it with scientific studies and in time generate an entire industry based on nothing more than an assumption which was never certain to begin with, should come as no surprise. We see it in the financial industry where dot com and real estate bubbles are believed in whole heartedly time and again until they inevitably do the unthinkable and explode. These myths are originated and perpetuated by those who stand to gain from them the most. Even when the falseness of their underlying assumptions is staring them in the face, people who have believed long enough and invested themselves deeply enough in the myth have an uncanny ability to turn the other cheek...until it's too late.

So what are the "dissidents" saying about HIV and AIDS?

One individual often credited with first questioning the connection between HIV and AIDS is Dr. Peter Duesberg. Dr. Duesberg is a tenured professor of molecular and cell biology at the University of California, Berkley, and he isolated the first cancer gene through his work on retroviruses in 1970. On his website, www.deusberg.com, you will find an extremely impressive biography and review of his challenge to the hypothesis that HIV causes AIDS, for which he paid a hefty price of being ostracized by the mainstream scientific community for standing by his convictions. In time, however, his views were supported by other prominent scientists, including the 1993 winner of the Nobel Prize for Chemistry, Dr. Kary Mullis.

Dr. Duesberg and Dr. Mullis, among others, believe that HIV is a harmless virus. No other known virus has the ability to behave as HIV is credited with behaving: at first the virus's behavior is typical with an initial infection triggering a fever, followed by development of antibodies and suppression of the virus by the immune system within a few days. But for HIV to come back after a decade or more of inactivity and somehow destroy the host's immune system remains, to this day, an unproven hypothesis. Despite billions of dollars of research funding, there is no proven mechanism of action by which HIV destroys T-cells (the latest hypothesis being that HIV stimulates immune cell "apoptosis," which is a natural process of cell suicide that occurs with all cells in the body). Furthermore, the behavior of the spread of AIDS has never followed the "pandemic" pattern of a viral spread, though the changing CDC definitions in 1987 and 1992 helped it appear that way.

Deusberg points out far more likely explanations for AIDS cases that are specific to geographic, cultural, and economic conditions of those afflicted. For example, widespread malnutrition in Africa especially with respect to animal protein and fat and adequate micronutrient availability (flour and starch are the primary "filler foods" in terms of calories per-dollar) is a known cause of many AIDS indicator diseases. Yet if immunity is low enough, the blame is automatically shifted to HIV. Given the importance of a balanced diet that includes APF and the countless ways nutrition supports our health and fights off disease, it's easy to see how those living on nutritionally limited diets would be susceptible to the diseases classified under AIDS.

As mentioned, AIDS is essentially an umbrella term for 29 separate diseases that occur in people who also have a certain low level of immunity. These "indicator diseases" include two that are particularly redundant and absurd; "HIV wasting disease" and low immunity in and of themselves! If you are an otherwise healthy person with no issues whatsoever, and your CD4*T cell count (a measure of your immune system) is below 200 cells per microliter, then you have AIDS and by definition, you're HIV positive!

All of the correlative studies linking HIV and AIDS (since there have been no *definitive* ones) among cohorts have alternative, more realistic explanations within those cohorts which Dr. Deusberg and others have highlighted in their research. These include malnutrition in poverty stricken countries, exact correlations between non random groups of AIDS sufferers and toxic recreational drug use within those groups, and the toxicity of HIV treatment itself. Drugs used in AIDS treatment were developed and circulated beginning in the late 80s and could have easily created the self-fulfilling prophecy that HIV infection leads to the deterioration of one's health and even death.

In a paper published in 2003 in the Journal of Bioscience by Peter Duesberg, Claus Koehnlein, and David Rasnick, titled *"The Chemical Bases of the Various AIDS Epidemics: Recreational Drugs, Anti-viral Chemotherapy and Malnutrition,"* (available at www.duesberg.com) the authors point out that there were many paradoxes within the virus-AIDS hypothesis that had not yet been resolved. These include (quoting directly from their paper) the following: "Why is there no HIV in AIDS patients, only antibodies against it? Why would HIV take 10 years from infection to AIDS? Why is AIDS not self limiting via antiviral immunity? Why is there no vaccine against AIDS? Why is AIDS in the US and Europe not random like other viral epidemics? Why is AIDS not contagious? Why would only HIV carriers get AIDS who use either recreational or anti-HIV drugs or are subject to malnutrition? **Why is the mortality of HIV-antibody-positives treated with anti-HIV drugs 7-9%, but that of all (mostly untreated) HIV-positives globally is only 1-4%?"** The Journal of Bioscience is a well established, highly regarded, peer reviewed scientific journal, and the authors of this paper have earned their credibility. Personally, I find it hard to see how people can fully dismiss these questions (posed two decades *after* HIV became the commonly accepted cause of AIDS) without at least considering their scientific validity.

    I don't want to go into this too deeply but would encourage anyone interested to visit Dr. Peter Duesberg's website to read more. What seems like a fail-safe thing to do, however, (again, this is NOT professional medical advice) is that if you are HIV positive or are suffering from any of the AIDS indicator diseases and wish to recover your health, begin shifting to the natural diet and lifestyle. If the degree of the illness is severe and chemotherapy or extremely toxic anti retroviral medications are in use, at least use them while adhering as best you can to the NDL.

    By reducing the acid load in your body, moving and oxygenating your blood everyday with moderate exercise, eating whole foods and digesting them efficiently, you'll begin to build your natural body strength back. By balancing your meals, taking advantage of the hunger cycles and following your hunger, you'll gain the strength to fight off whatever "indicator" disease has taken hold and also better tolerate and eliminate the toxicity of medications.

In impoverished societies where nutrition is extremely poor and animal protein is extremely scarce due to its high price, I believe foreign aid for programs that help AIDS patients need to focus on increasing availability of quality animal foods and vegetables in local diets. If some of the money spent on medication was re-directed towards nutrition and making healing meals based on the natural diet available, it stands to reason that we would see huge changes in the health and well being of AIDS sufferers worldwide.

## ALCOHOLISM AND ADDICTIONS

There are few bigger demons than the demons of addiction. Like other chronic illnesses, once addiction takes hold it is a self-perpetuating cycle that builds momentum over time. To overcome an addiction, one must understand the underlying cause and what triggered it. This cause almost always takes the form of an emotional or spiritual emptiness. Sometimes the emptiness wasn't there at first but the substance brought it on. Other times it was there to begin with and the substance provided an escape. Either way, just as with chronic depression, one must decide at some point to rally everything in their power to make a complete and lasting change in their lives.

Like depression, addictions cannot be overcome alone. There is a reason that Alcoholics Anonymous (AA) and drug rehab centers exist; not because people are weak and can't do it by themselves but because people are people; when serious problems enter our lives we all need help and love and support from others. We need to know we're not alone. We need the guidance of those who have been in our shoes and can steer us back, just as someone else guided them back.

Addictions are temporary escapes from darkness. They fill the areas in our lives that are lacking physically and/or emotionally and give us a false sense of elevation that inevitably worsens that which it hides. Fighting these demons cannot be done alone and will not succeed in the presence of "enablers"...friends or acquaintances who suffer from the same addictions but who lack the will to fight and want to pull you down with them.

Addictions ruin lives and strip us of the gifts we have to give the world. In taking that first step by making a firm commitment to enter a prolonged fight with our addictions (and all other chronic disease for that matter), we acknowledge that we do have gifts and limitless potential to help others and leave this world better than we found it. To take on the demons of addiction is the first step on the most noble of paths: a path towards the belief in goodness.

The first step in overcoming alcoholism or other addiction is extricating oneself from the geographic/social context of your addiction. Move. If you have friends/enablers to whom you feel obligated to explain your move, be as truthful and concise as possible: "I'm moving because I need to stop drinking/doing drugs/etc. so I can regain my health and a positive direction in life." Put it in writing if that's easier. Friends might do everything in their power to keep you, but if they're real friends, they'll respect you and perhaps you'll even inspire them to do the same.

The next step is to ask healthy, positive people you can trust (family, friends, and/or support groups) for help. Do this as soon as you move, or set it up beforehand. There is no reason to fight a battle alone if help is available (and as mentioned, it's almost always necessary). Ask them to support you in your effort to follow the natural diet and lifestyle, to accompany you on outdoor activities and adventures and to do interesting things every day and night so you're not alone. Above all, try to find an outlet that is mentally stimulating and nourishing to the soul to supplant the addiction. Perhaps reading or writing poetry or keeping a journal of your inner thoughts and feelings, learning about a religion or how to play an instrument. By somehow expressing the problems within, you can separate them from your true self and control them. Channel yourself into something positive that you can share with others, or find something that you feel is worthwhile volunteering for.

While addictions usually fill a spiritual void, don't forget that there is also a chemical and physical side to them as well. By eating healthy, balanced meals and maintaining a natural circadian rhythm in your daily life, you can help bring your physical body back into balance and all cravings, including those of your addictions will dissipate as well. When the body has what it needs nutritionally, the spirit is strengthened as well.

Above all, hold fast to your commitment. If you fall, get up and try again. Never stop trying. Believe in yourself and open your heart to the world.

## ARTHRITIS

Arthritis is an inflammation of the joints brought on by tight muscles and ligaments and an overly acidic body. As with other chronic illnesses I believe the key to avoiding and reversing arthritis is by living naturally and avoiding acid-producing and toxic substances such as alcohol, drugs, and excessive medications.

Daily exercise will oxygenate and rid the body of toxic acid-build up and daily whole-body stretching will help loosen and relax muscles and ligaments. This should be undertaken in a very moderate and consistent manner to avoid stretch injuries.

Most important, the NDL with an emphasis on leafy greens, seaweed, and deeply alkalizing vegetables will drastically reduce the body's propensity toward inflammation by providing the nutrients (especially minerals such as magnesium and potassium) necessary to relax the muscles that are constantly tight and pulling on the joints. Like many other illnesses, arthritis is an overly yin or acidic condition and by alkalizing the body and shifting towards the natural diet and lifestyle, arthritis symptoms will dissipate and the body will heal.

## CANCER

There are about 200 different types of cancer, but all cancers are characterized by abnormal cell growth and subsequent invasion of that growth into other parts of the body. Cancer is thought to be caused by damage to genes and cells by excess acid, insufficient oxygen, exposure to toxic chemicals, radiation, or viral infections.

A healthy environment for our cells is one that is oxygen rich and slightly alkaline. Such an environment is extremely inhospitable to viruses and pathogenic organisms, and toxins are quickly neutralized and disposed of. Cancer cells cannot exist in richly oxygenated, alkaline environments. This was hypothesized by Dr. Otto Warburg, shortly after winning the Nobel Prize for Medicine in 1931. In his words;

"Cancer, above all other diseases, has countless secondary causes. But, even for cancer, there is only one primary cause.

Summarized in a few words, the prime cause of cancer is the replacement of the respiration of oxygen in normal body cells by a fermentation of sugar..."

Today it is widely accepted that cancer cells differ from healthy cells in that they do indeed metabolize sugar for energy anaerobically (without oxygen) as Warburg said. However, there are many risk factors for cancer besides acid which include a long list of toxic chemicals as well as radiation.

To reduce your risk of cancer or to help recover from it, it's essential to adhere to the NDL and completely eliminate habits/substances that may have caused the cancer to begin with, such as smoking, alcohol, or drugs. Oxygenating the blood and lowering acid build up through the natural diet and increasing circulation by exercising daily to the extent possible will maximize your chances of successfully fighting cancer or avoiding it to begin with.

## CROHN'S DISEASE AND IRRITABLE BOWEL SYNDROME (IBS)

Irritable Bowel Syndrome (IBS) and Crohn's disease both refer to a chronic inflammatory condition of the small and large intestines that presents with frequent and often extreme bouts of diarrhea. Symptoms tend to flare up and dissipate and flare up again. The cause of IBS and Crohn's is uncertain, but I see it simply as chronic gastritis shifted to the lower intestines. The inflammation could be bacterial, fungal, or viral in origin. As in upper GI gastritis, inflammation of the small intestine and/or large intestine results in increased porosity of those membranes, which in turn allows a rapid osmotic diffusion of water across the intestinal wall, causing diarrhea and an inability to absorb nutrients.

In understanding Crohn's and IBS, it's helpful to understand the concept of osmotic diffusion across a semipermeable membrane. The entire human body is filled with fluids separated by semi-permeable membranes that absorb and secreting substances in a both *passive* and *active* manner. Small molecules and minerals such as water, sodium and potassium often cross membranes in a *passive* manner by naturally flowing, or diffusing across the membrane from the side of high concentration to the side of low concentration. Increasing or decreasing the concentration of fluid on a given side of a semipermeable membrane influences the direction of diffusion. This type of diffusion is called *osmosis*.

Pure water is itself a very dense fluid. When particles are added to water, such as salt or sugar, they dissolve and have the effect of pushing water molecules out of their tight, dense arrangement, making the resulting fluid less dense. If this solution is separated from pure distilled water by a semi-permeable membrane (that allows water molecules through but nothing else), then water molecules will dissolve across the membrane into the water with the dissolved salt or sugar. This will continue until the pressure on both sides has equalized.

## Osmosis

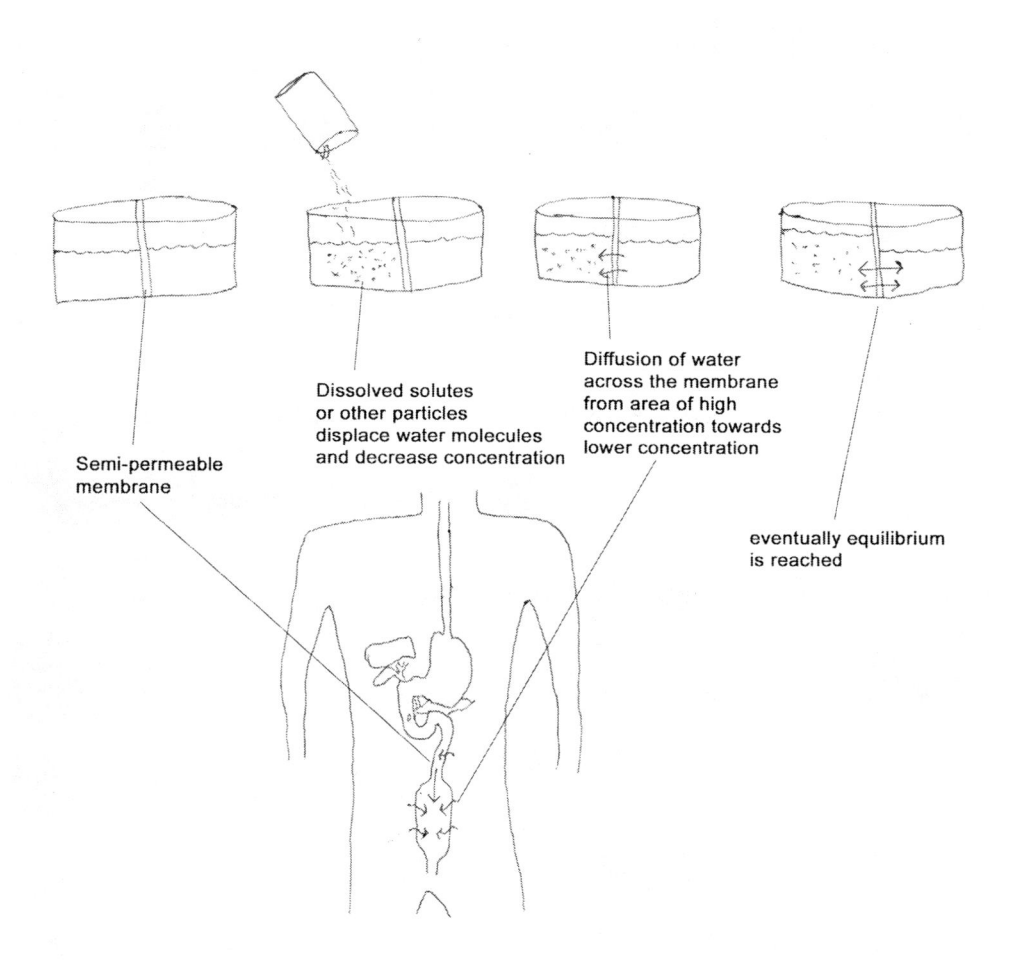

Semi-permeable membrane

Dissolved solutes or other particles displace water molecules and decrease concentration

Diffusion of water across the membrane from area of high concentration towards lower concentration

eventually equilibrium is reached

*Osmotic diffusion across semi-permeable membranes*

In cases of acute bacterial overgrowth causing inflammation in the bowels, this cascade of inflammation and osmotic diffusion of water from the blood across the intestinal wall causing diarrhea is a natural, beneficial way of ridding the intestines of harmful bacterial or yeast overgrowth. However, if the inflammation becomes chronic, the constant diarrhea starves the body of nutrients and leads to a gradual wasting away.

The NDL can heal Crohn's and IBS over time by increasing digestive power with the stimulation of AD, which will break down food for more rapid absorption before it has time to pass down into the lower intestines and ferment and/or trigger diarrhea. In addition, minerals and nutrients absorbed into the blood help retain a higher blood osmolality, which helps to balance the osmotic difference across the gastrointestinal tract, keeping water in the blood and absorbing more nutrients as well.

Over time, well digested, balanced meals (being broken down in the duodenal cauldron of Active Digestion) can both provide nutrients for healing and slowly re-establish the beneficial flora in the lower GI tract, which are necessary to producing the antibacterial, antiviral, antiinflammatory and immune-regulating compounds that ultimately re-balance the body and heal Crohn's and IBS.

## DEPRESSION

To reiterate what I mentioned in the beginning of this chapter, depression can be a very complex and challenging illness, and I don't want to oversimplify this or any other illness, but only offer a few ideas that might be helpful.

Everyone has experienced depression at some point or other in their lives, and others deal with levels of chronic depression that have all but completely destroyed them. Like all chronic diseases, depression is a self-perpetuating cycle that requires a concerted effort to break free from. There can be many triggers of chronic depression, both physical and emotional, but as depression takes hold, it saps the person of the motivation to live naturally; to eat right and exercise every day, and to engage in regular social activities. Lack of motivation prolongs and deepens their depressed state.

To break the cycle of depression, one must understand that aside from the emotional or physical trigger, depression (especially extreme depression) is very much a state of chemistry in the body, perpetuated by toxins or nutritional deficiencies. Often people with depression will find relief through intoxication with drugs and/or alcohol. Unfortunately, this only exacerbates the nutritional imbalance in their bodies, leaching important nutrients like magnesium and potassium as well as vitamins and hormones. The combined effect further impairs one's psyche and well-being.

Because depression can be so deeply incapacitating, recovering from it is an uphill battle that's rarely accomplished alone. Those afflicted must find it in themselves to leave the toxic lifestyle and toxic relationships that have caused or perpetuated their depression and seek out the love and support of a healthier tribe. Being around people who are healthy, understanding, and positive, and taking baby steps towards maintaining the natural diet and lifestyle can help one escape the powerful grasp of chronic depression. Focus particularly on part five of chapter five; "Maintaining a physically and mentally active lifestyle." Sunshine has a well known and direct effect on mood along with exercise, so getting outside every day and being active, and finding and cultivating interests that stimulate you mentally are key factors in recovery.

Conquering depression is like beating cancer; it is no less serious and no less intense. It's a battle that can be a lifelong dedication, but the more resolved one is to understand it and the more one believes in his or her worth and potential to someday help others, then recovery is possible. The key is to stay active and not dwell on the past. We cannot change what happened to us or what we did, but we can change how we live now and how we move forward into the future. If depression comes from a loss of control or a giving up, then we need to fight to regain control one small step at a time.

The title of the short poem below by William Henley (written in 1875 at age 25, in the hospital bed after his leg was amputated due to tuberculosis) was also the title of a movie about Nelson Mandela's rise from imprisonment to the presidency in post-apartheid South Africa. It seems appropriate for this section on overcoming depression. After all, depression is one illness common to all others. The battle for health is a battle we fight with the help of others, but at times we must also fight alone.

*Invictus*

*(Latin for "Undefeated")*

*Out of the night that covers me,*
*Black as the pit from pole to pole,*
*I thank whatever gods may be*
*For my unconquerable soul.*

*In the fell clutch of circumstance*
*I have not winced nor cried aloud.*
*Under the bludgeonings of chance*
*My head is bloody, but unbowed.*

*Beyond this place of wrath and tears*
*Looms but the Horror of the shade,*
*And yet the menace of the years*
*Finds, and shall find me, unafraid.*

*It matters not how strait the gate,*
*How charged with punishments the scroll.*
*I am the master of my fate:*
*I am the captain of my soul*

## TYPE II DIABETES

Type 2 diabetes is the result of a decrease in effectiveness of the hormone *insulin*. Since insulin is responsible for signaling the cells of the body to accept sugar, this resistance to insulin results in elevated levels of blood sugar and a host of symptoms that may include extreme thirst, extreme hunger (since cells aren't getting the glucose they need to produce energy), fatigue, irritability, excessive urination, fainting and stroke, and many other symptoms. According to a report dated June 2008 from the National Institute of Health, about 23.6 million Americans had Type 2 Diabetes and another 58 million were pre-diabetic, meaning they're prone to develop Type 2 Diabetes because of their current health condition and lifestyle.

There are many conditions associated with insulin resistance and Type 2 Diabetes, including obesity and problems with the eyes, heart, brain, feet, and nerves. But at the cellular level all these conditions relate to cells of the body saying "no" to insulin and therefore saying "no" to more sugar entering the cells.

Now, why would a cell say "no" to sugar? I believe it's because of a pH imbalance within the cells themselves. Recall that acid is a byproduct of cellular metabolism. If the acid produced by cells is not being buffered within the cell by proteins or disposed of quickly enough (into the blood and ultimately through the lungs, feces, or urine), the pH within the cell will drop. This poses an enormous risk to the survivability of the cell since a drop in the pH inside a cell will denature proteins that keep the cell functioning and eventually even denature DNA itself which could lead to cancer or death.

To keep this from happening, the cells become insulin resistant (by way of an acid-triggered cascade), refusing to let more sugar in that will otherwise get metabolized and increase the acidity of the cell (decrease the pH) to deadly levels. In fact there is a natural mechanism of cell-death within the body called *apoptosis* in which a cell will have lived out its useful lifespan or becomes infected and then kills itself before mutating into something potentially harmful to the body as a whole. This process of apoptosis is apparently dependent on acidification of the cell (Gottlieb, R.A. "Cell Acidification in Apoptosis" Apoptosis 1:1).

While there could be many possible ways for acid build-up within cells to trigger a cascade by which proteins no longer respond to insulin, from an evolutionary point of view this would be an entirely natural mechanism of self-preservation. Excessive acid inside cells would lead to much worse, irreversible problems and eventually death.

Diabetes, therefore, is not so much a disease as it is a warning to exercise more and get back to a natural diet that minimizes acidity and increases the alkalinity and acid-buffering capacity of the body. It's common knowledge that diabetes (Type II, at least) is a disease that develops through a diet high in refined sugars and starches. Months or years of unnaturally high doses of sugar in modern-day meals and snacks which lack their whole food micronutrient alkalizing and acid buffering components take a toll on the pH balance of the intracellular environment. To protect themselves, the cells begin simply refusing sugar, *for good reason.*

By steering towards the NDL, the symptoms of diabetes can be mitigated and in some cases reversed. Balanced meals of whole foods in a circadian eating cycle will regulate the body and dispose of cravings that result in "quick fixes" of unnatural and high Glycemic Index foods. The "Glycemic Index," or GI, refers to the rate at which different sources of carbohydrates break down into sugar and enter the blood stream. High GI foods such as refined flour or table sugar provide a rapid dose of sugar to the blood which is problematic for diabetics, while low GI foods provide a steady supply of blood sugar without the dangerous "spike" that's often followed by a "crash" in blood sugar. Balanced meals that include APF and wholesome carbohydrates are digested slowly and provide the body with a constant supply of nutrients for hours to come. Getting active with daily exercise will oxygenate the blood and regulate acidity as well, easing the burden of acid build-up within cells and over time minimizing or even eliminating the symptoms of diabetes.

# MONONUCLEOSIS

*Mononucleosis*, or "Mono," is a contagious illness caused by an infection of the Epstein-Barr virus. The virus takes hold when the individual's immune system is weak due to poor diet, stimulants, and lack of sleep (conditions that can be brought on by stressful, high work load environments or self inflicted by individual standards of achievement) and is known for leaving its host completely "wiped out" for weeks on end. An hour or two of "normal" energy a day is the most many people with this illness can muster, and even then it's a hazy and groggy state of affairs.

Having suffered from both chronic fatigue symptoms and Mononucleosis I can say that the symptoms on bad days with CFS and a normal day with Mono are very similar. My own theory for the cause of fatigue in mono (since the exact mechanism by which the Epstein-Barr virus causes mono symptoms is unknown) is the same as in CFS; the virus causes inflammation of the stomach through which stomach acid leaks into the blood. This throws off the sensitive alkaline blood pH, leading to a reduced oxygen carrying capacity of blood and the systemic build up of acid. The overall effect is total body weakness and malaise. In addition, the inflamed stomach results in impaired digestion and food is less efficiently broken down and absorbed, keeping the body weak.

Those suffering with mononucleosis will do well to follow the natural diet and focus on balanced meals that shift the digestive burden from the stomach and trigger Active Digestion. Unlike the CFS sufferer, those with Mono do not necessarily lack healthy intestinal flora, and by eating balanced meals on a circadian regimen, and getting outside and moving around a little every day to help oxygenate the blood, you can recover from mono within weeks instead of months.

APF and greens are powerful parts of the diet when recovering from Mono. Remember that in during Mono, the stomach is inflamed and digestion is compromised, so eat tender, organic meats and eat when hungry. Snack on fruits and adhere in other respects to the natural diet and lifestyle for a quick recovery...

## OBESITY

Obese people live in a state of constant hunger because they are starving nutritionally. The natural diet and lifestyle solves this problem by providing an abundance of nutrients and oxygenating the body every day with moderate exercise. When the body is given the nutrients it needs and the blood is oxygenated, hunger cravings give way to increased energy and satisfaction with each meal. By adhering to the NDL, obese people will fall back into their natural, healthy body weight and as a result will shed other problems such as depression and low self esteem along the way. However, it's also important to acknowledge that while losing weight makes you thinner, it doesn't magically solve all other problems in life. Many overweight people believe that if they could just be thin, their lives would be perfect but that is a delusion. While it's certainly an important piece of the puzzle and decreases the risk of other illnesses such as Type 2 Diabetes, obesity *can* be a symptom of psychological issues such as depression. Since the NDL addresses health issues from nearly every angle, weight loss within the broader context of the NDL is far more effective than simply focusing on losing weight alone.

## HEALING FROM INJURIES

Having been a competitive athlete for most of my life, I've had plenty of experience with all kinds of injuries including Iliotibial Band Syndrome (ITBS), plantar fasciitis, runner's knee, and many more. Healing from all of these injuries can be greatly facilitated by adopting a natural diet and lifestyle.

Depending on the severity of the injury, it's tempting to either lay off exercise completely or to ignore the injury until it gets so bad that you have to lay off exercises completely. What I've learned over the years is that by staying active within one's comfort zone, injuries heal much faster. For example, if you have runner's knee or ITBS, not exercising at all isn't the answer. The answer is to do what you can everyday and stop BEFORE you feel pain, even if what you can do is minimal. By moving to the extent that you comfortably can, you keep blood circulating which carries off acid and toxins from the site of injury while introducing healing oxygen and nutrients. Some parts of the body, including our knees and joints, actually depend on movement and light compression to circulate nutrients and heal. Think of our evolution as a species – unless our injuries were severe, we kept moving to the extent we could because we had to. But the key was and remains: avoid pain! Pain is the obvious sign that more damage than healing is being done.

I had a six month bout with ITBS which I finally ended through daily light running and "passive" stretching within my comfort zone. By "passive" stretching I mean stretching with virtually no exertion. The idea is to not aggravate any injured or damaged tissues but to gradually and carefully lengthen the muscle and tendons to relieve tightness and allow for healing and inflammation to subside. By doing light, passive stretching before, during, and after exercise every day, I was able to gradually lengthen my IT band which relieved the friction, damage, and inflammation. The distance of my runs gradually increased until the problem disappeared altogether within a few weeks, but the key was consistency and always staying within my comfort zone.

People tend to underestimate the role of diet in healing sports-related or overuse injuries, but I believe a natural, alkalizing diet can make a night or day difference when it comes to healing injuries. One's blood is constantly bathing injured tissues and your blood is rich in oxygen and healing nutrients, everything will heal faster than if your blood lacks the nutrients and alkalinity to heal and ward off inflammation.

## CONCLUSION

Drugs and medications have allayed many symptoms but have not provided cures to most chronic illnesses and in my opinion probably never will. How can anything take the place of the abundance of nutrients in whole foods being efficiently digested and absorbed? What drug can take the place of stretching, exercise, fresh air, and sunlight on a daily basis?

For millions of years, humanity has evolved without much of what we put in our bodies today – from the synthesized chemical compounds we call medicine to the prevalence of cheap alcohol, refined and processed foods, and meats of animals raised in toxic environments. When these foods are consumed on a daily basis for years on end, the body pays a price.

As the global monetary culture has given rise to an abundance of goods and services, it has become easier to lose sight of the simple things that keep us alive and well: positive relationships, foods that balance and energize, and activities that engage us mentally and physically. The medical industry has convinced a lot of people that healing doesn't require work; indeed work is the last thing most people want to do. But if there's one thing I want the reader to come away with after reading this book, it's that you CAN overcome chronic illness...by arming yourself with knowledge and believing in yourself (even if doctors or those around you don't) and the good that you have to offer and to experience by working towards a healing. It is important to never give up, despite the set-backs and slips. By shifting back to our natural diet and maximizing digestive power in the ways I've described in this guide, I believe people can avoid and overcome most of the chronic diseases that plague 21st century society.

Humans have the ability to be healthy and happy. By living simpler, physically active, and self-responsible lives, ours will become a healthier and more sustainable world.

**About the Author:**

Jonathan "Troy" Hull was born in Nairobi, Kenya, in 1979 and raised overseas in Greece, Indonesia, and Mexico City before attending The Putney School in Putney, Vermont. While living overseas his family bought a house in central Maine which became home. Troy went on to attend Vassar College where he designed an independent major in Ethnobotany stemming from an interest in tropical forest conservation, and ran competitively on the cross country team before graduating in 2002. He has owned and operated a home renovation business for the past 8 years and coached a high school track team while living in Maine. In college, Troy contracted a stomach virus that left him with inexplicable fatigue and triggered his interest in health and chronic illness. He currently lives in Maine and remains a competitive distance runner, father, and business owner.

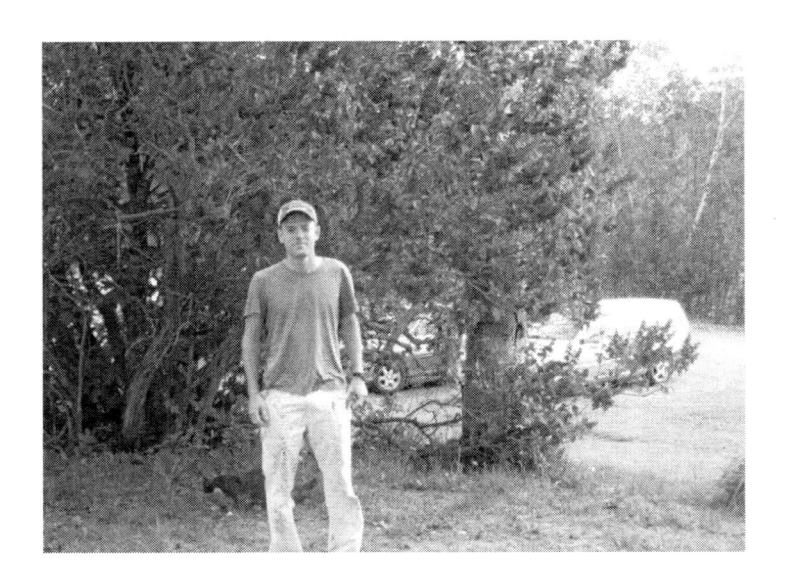